WELLNESS
BY THE
NUMBERS

WELLNESS BY THE NUMBERS

Understanding and Interpreting
American Health Statistics

JACQUELINE KLOSEK

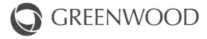 GREENWOOD

AN IMPRINT OF ABC-CLIO, LLC
Santa Barbara, California • Denver, Colorado • Oxford, England

Library of Congress Cataloging-in-Publication Data

Klosek, Jacqueline, 1972-
   Wellness by the numbers : understanding and interpreting American health statistics / Jacqueline Klosek.
      pages cm
   Includes bibliographical references.
   ISBN 978-1-61069-963-1 (hardback) — ISBN 978-1-61069-964-8 (e-book)
1. Health status indicators—United States.   2. Diseases—United States—Statistics.   3. United States—Statistics, Medical.   I. Title.
   RA407.3.K53 2015
   614.4'2—dc23   2014040151

ISBN: 978-1-61069-963-1
EISBN: 978-1-61069-964-8

19 18 17 16 15   1 2 3 4 5

This book is also available on the World Wide Web as an eBook.
Visit www.abc-clio.com for details.

Greenwood
An Imprint of ABC-CLIO, LLC

ABC-CLIO, LLC
130 Cremona Drive, P.O. Box 1911
Santa Barbara, California 93116-1911

This book is printed on acid-free paper ∞

Manufactured in the United States of America

This book is dedicated to my darling daughter Kayla Emerson Lozinski. You are the ultimate source of light, love, and inspiration. I love you more than words can say. May you always be blessed with the best of health.

CONTENTS

INTRODUCTION

Recently, the amount of money that Americans spend on health care exceeded $3.8 trillion.[1] This astonishing figure demonstrates the high value that Americans place on good health—and the struggles that we are facing in achieving good health. Individuals are increasingly aware that with good health, they can feel better, look better, and live longer. Across the country, people are devoting time to reading health-related information, all in an effort to try to determine how to protect themselves from diseases, to uncover the latest ways to lose weight, and to identify the best diets that will help their bodies be stronger and live longer.

The media has responded to the concerns that we have about health optimization and today, we have incredible access to a deluge of health-related information. Magazines, books, television shows, websites, mobile applications, and social media services are all brimming with information about various health and medical information. And, yet, while there is this abundance of information available for consumption, it can be difficult for health care consumers to sort through what information is accurate, current, and

---

[1] Dan Muro, "Annual U.S. Healthcare Spending Hits $3.8 Trillion," Forbes, February 2, 2014, http://www.forbes.com/sites/danmunro/2014/02/02/annual-u-s-healthcare-spending-hits-3-8-trillion.

credible. The best health information is based on scientific research, but occasionally scientific evidence can be misunderstood or misinterpreted by those reporting on it. Even worse, those with vested interests can sometimes purposefully mischaracterize research findings in order to serve their own purposes.

The goal of *Wellness by the Numbers: Understanding and Interpreting American Health Statistics* is to provide clear and concise information about certain key health issues. This book commences with a discussion on strategies for locating health-related information online and evaluating that information. The book then explores a number of key health topics, from maladies including various types of cancers, to discussions of topics that might lead to improved health, such as physical exercise and vitamin supplementation. Each section of the book defines and discusses one particular health indicator and then presents key data regarding that issue. Finally, each section concludes with discussion questions for further thought, investigation, and consideration.

ACKNOWLEDGMENTS

I gratefully acknowledge the valuable assistance of Amanda Kontor, Carly Long, and Kevin Holton.

LOCATING ACCURATE AND CURRENT DATA ON HEALTH-RELATED INFORMATION ONLINE

UNDERSTANDING WEB-BASED HEALTH-RELATED INFORMATION

Health-related information is easily accessible with today's technology; however, certain questions should be asked to evaluate the accuracy and currency of the provided information. Individuals should also recognize that determining the accuracy of health-related information can be difficult at times, even with credible sources of information. Conflicting information or differences of expert opinion may be found when a topic is newly researched, not yet fully understood, or can be treated in various ways. Therefore, it is always important to consult with an individual's medical practitioner before making any health-related decisions based on information that is found on the Internet. Yet, there are several ways to get a good understanding of health-related topics and to ensure that the information is credible. When relying on information from the Internet, individuals should ask the five Ws: who, what, when, where, and why.

HOW TO LOCATE ACCURATE AND CURRENT DATA

Determining who has posted the health information is an easy way to establish the accuracy of a site. Most websites will list the authors of the information, or the sponsors that provided the information. If no author or sponsor is provided, individuals can look for an "About" link to learn more about the purpose of the website and if the providers are credible. Additionally, examining the website URL can give an idea of whether the information is accurate. URLs that end in .gov are government-sponsored sites and can be trusted. URLs that end in .edu are educational institution sites and can be trusted, except when it is a personal page. URLs that end in .org are noncommercial organization sites and do not guarantee authorization, as they may provide false or biased information. URLs that end in .com are commercial organization sites and are the least trustworthy sites; however, hospitals may obtain a .com URL, so there are exceptions in verifying the accuracy of .com sites. By learning who has posted the health information, individuals can determine how the site is funded and if this factor affects the content that is provided. If the information was not posted by a reliable health-related source or known health organization, individuals can look for whether the information was reviewed by a medical expert or doctor. The credentials of the source may also be examined to determine whether the source has the required expertise to provide health-related information. If the information has undergone peer review, that further enhances the accuracy of the information. Additionally, contact information of the source, which is usually located at the bottom of the page, also enhances the accuracy of the information.

What the information says is also important in determining accuracy and currency. When reading through the information, individuals should make sure that proper grammar and punctuation are used. Sensational writing styles should be avoided. Also, information should not appear to be opinion based. All facts and statistics should be cited and refer to an original scientific study or medical expert.

Determining when the information was originally posted or last reviewed will help ensure the currency of the information. Health information changes constantly, as researchers are continuously making new health-related discoveries that are being posted across the Internet. Individuals should check the date of when the information was originally posted or last reviewed, which is usually provided at the bottom of the page. If this information is not provided, they should look for the copyright line, which informs when the original information was posted. Individuals should try to find health-related information that was reviewed within the past year to ensure its currency. Another way to check the currency of the information is to click on links that are provided on the page to ensure that they are not broken links, as that can signify that the site is not current.

Determining where the information comes from will help ensure accuracy. If the information does not come directly from the site publisher, references should be listed to describe the evidence that the material is based on. For example, educational institutions or hospital sites may acknowledge specific health information that was reposted from medical journals or other scientific research. Social media sites may provide a small portion of information; however, they should have links that will direct individuals to the full-length article, where they can determine who originally posted the information and when it was originally posted. Special tools can help authenticate social media sites, such as the U.S. federal government's site, www.usa.gov/Contact/verify-social-media. shtml, which verifies social media accounts that claim to belong to federal agencies. Information that is supported by scientific studies or expert opinion must also be examined to further ensure accuracy. The original study should be examined to determine the study's methodology, size, focus, limitations, and so forth. For example, if a study has a small sample size, specific population, or many recognized weaknesses, its accuracy is lessened.

Determining why the site was created relates to figuring out who is posting the information, which will ensure the accuracy of the information. The purpose of the site can be learned in the "About" section of the site and will help individuals determine whether any bias may be used in the presentation of the information. All advertisements should be labeled. Also, look for "Privacy" links, as credible health sources should recognize the importance of protecting individual's privacy when regarding confidential health information.

CREDIBLE RESOURCES TO START WITH

Accurate and current health information can be easily found if research is started with certain credible resources. These sites are government sponsored, providing easily accessible information about the source, date, related links, etc. Examples include:

- www.cdc.gov: Sponsored by the Centers for Disease Control and Prevention
- www.who.int: Sponsored by the World Health Organization

- www.nlm.nih.gov/medlineplus/: Sponsored by the National Library of Medicine
- www.nih.gov: Sponsored by the National Institutes of Health
- www.healthfinder.gov: Sponsored by the Office of Disease Prevention and Health Promotion in the U.S. Department of Health and Human Services

1

ADHD

INTRODUCTION

Understanding ADHD

Attention deficit hyperactivity disorder (ADHD) is a relatively common childhood behavioral disorder that is characterized by inattention, hyperactivity, and impulsivity. There are three main subtypes of ADHD: predominantly hyperactive-impulsive, predominantly inattentive, and combined hyperactive-impulsive and inattentive. Combined hyperactive-impulsive and inattentive is the most prevalent type of ADHD in children. Subtypes are categorized by the prevalence of hyperactive-impulsive or inattentive symptoms.

Symptoms

The main symptoms of ADHD are severe and/or frequent inattention, hyperactivity, and impulsivity, each as further discussed below.

Symptoms categorized with inattention include:

- Distraction, forgetfulness, and inattentive to details
- Difficultly focusing on one task, switching tasks frequently
- Difficulty with organization and completion of tasks

- Trouble completing or turning in homework assignments
- Trouble listening, daydreaming
- Difficulty processing information as quickly and accurately as other
- Trouble following instruction

Symptoms categorized with hyperactivity include:

- Restlessness, constant movement
- Frequent talking
- Trouble sitting still
- Difficulty with quiet tasks

Symptoms categorized with impulsivity include:

- Impatience
- Acting without regard for consequences, inappropriate actions
- Interrupting conversation or tasks

Diagnosis

There is currently no single test that can diagnose ADHD. To be diagnosed with ADHD, a child must present severe symptoms for six or more months. Pediatricians or mental health specialists will first try to rule out other possible conditions that present with similar symptoms. A comprehensive evaluation will be completed to determine whether the child is suffering from undetected seizures, hearing or vision problems, learning disabilities, anxiety or depression, or significant environmental changes. In addition, professionals must consider the duration and frequency of the symptoms, the setting of the symptomatic behaviors, and how these behaviors impact the child's life.

Predominantly inattentive children may be overlooked, as they are often quiet and may seem as though they are paying attention to their work, but are not successfully getting any work completed. Additionally, children with predominantly hyperactive-impulsive symptoms may be overlooked as having emotional or disciplinary problems. Typically, teachers notice the symptoms first, followed by parents.

Contrary to the possibility of misdiagnosis, studies show increasing numbers of children are diagnosed with ADHD; however, the cause of this increase must still be researched.

In adults, a wider range of symptoms must be considered when being evaluated by a licensed mental health professional. The symptoms of ADHD must have begun in childhood and persisted throughout adulthood to be diagnosed. Rating scales, physical exams, and psychological tests may be used to determine diagnosis.

Additionally, ADHD may coexist with certain other disorders, including:

- Learning disabilities
- Oppositional defiant disorder
- Conduct disorder
- Anxiety and depression
- Bipolar disorder
- Tourette syndrome
- Sleep disorders
- Substance abuse

Risk Factors and Causation

ADHD is one of the most common childhood disorders, with the average age of onset being seven years old. Boys are four times more likely to have ADHD than girls. Approximately 9.0% of Americans age 13–18 are affected by ADHD. Additionally, an estimated 4.1% Americans age 18 years and older are affected each year.

Scientists are still researching the cause of ADHD. Current studies provide genetics as the most plausible cause, as children with a certain gene variations tend to have thinner brain tissue in areas linked to attention; however, the brain-tissue thickness and ADHD symptoms improved with age. Environmental factors, brain injuries, pregnancy complications, and nutrition are possible causes as well.

Treatment

While there is no cure for ADHD, the goal of treatment is to reduce symptoms of ADHD and improve functioning. Treatment options include medication, various types of psychotherapy, education, or a combination of treatments.

Stimulants, which produce a calming effect, are the most common medication used to treat ADHD. Many stimulant medications are available; however, nonstimulants are also available. Medication can come in various forms and each individual will react differently, so it is important to be monitored by a licensed professional. Most medication will reduce predominant hyperactivity-impulsive symptoms, while improving the ability to focus and listen. The most common side effects of stimulant medication includes a decreased appetite, sleep problems, and less often the development of sudden, repetitive movements known as tics. Other rare side effects are possible and must be discussed upon administration of the medication. Examples of approved medication include Adderall, Concerta, Dexedrine, and Ritalin. Due to interaction with other medicines, adults must consult a professional to determine which medications are approved for them. In certain cases, adults may be administered antidepressants.

Various types of psychotherapy are available to help individuals with ADHD. Behavioral therapy aims to help change behavior with the use of reinforcements and may include assistance in organization and completion of tasks. Monitoring one's behavior and acquiring social skills are other learned features of behavioral therapy.

With treatment, most individuals with ADHD can be successful. Researchers are currently studying other effective methods of treatment and exploring the use of new tools, such as brain imaging, to gain a better understanding of ADHD.

DATA AND ANALYSES

Data

Table 1.1 Emergency Department (ED) Visits Related to Attention Deficit Hyperactivity Disorder (ADHD) Stimulant Medications by Age Group: 2005 and 2010

Age group	2005 ED visits related to ADHD medication	2010 ED visits related to ADHD medication
Aged 5 to 11	3,322	3,791
Aged 12 to 17	2,702	3,461
Aged 18 to 25	2,131	8,148
Aged 26 to 34	1,754	6,094
Aged 35 or older	2,519	7,957

Source: Substance Abuse and Mental Health Services Administration. 2013. "Emergency department visits involving attention deficit/hyperactivity disorder stimulant medications." Center for Behavioral Health Statistics and Quality. Retrieved from: http://www.samhsa.gov/data/2k13/dawn073/sr073-add-adhd-medications.htm

Analysis

ADHD is often treated with stimulant medication. When used correctly, stimulant medications can improve ADHD symptoms; however, there is also the risk of negative side effects such as cardiovascular or psychiatric problems. Table 1.1 shows that there were a total of 17,865 more emergency department visits related to this medication in 2010 than 2005. The majority of increased visits were among adults 18 years and older. Of these visits, there was a severe increase in those that were caused by nonmedical use of the medication. From 2005 to 2010, there were a total of 10,373 more visits related to nonmedical use. The medication may be misused to suppress appetite, enhance focus, or cause feelings of happiness. By continuing to monitor the relation of emergency department visits to nonmedical use of stimulant medications, interventions can be developed and applied to decrease the number of ED visits in future years.

Data

Table 1.2 Percentage of Children Aged 5–17 Ever Diagnosed with ADHD: Division by Gender From 1998 to 2009

Years studied	Males diagnosed with ADHD	Females diagnosed with ADHD
1998–2000	9.9%	3.6%
2001–2003	10.7%	4.1%
2004–2006	11.4%	4.6%
2007–2009	12.3%	5.5%

Source: Akinbami, L., Liu, X., Pastor, P., & Reuben, C. 2011. "Attention deficit hyperactivity disorder among children aged 5–17 years in the United States, 1998–2009." Centers for Disease Control and Prevention. Retrieved from: http://www.cdc.gov/nchs/data/databriefs/db70.htm

Analysis

Typically, boys are four times more likely than girls to be diagnosed with ADHD. Table 1.2 details overall diagnoses between males and females aged 5–17 between the years of 1998 and 2009. Results support the higher risk factor of ADHD in males, as well as the increasing number of diagnoses.

DISCUSSION QUESTIONS

1. ADHD stimulant medication has led to increased number of emergency department visits. What are possible causes for this?
2. The prevalence of ADHD is increasing. In your opinion, what is the cause of the increase in ADHD diagnosis? Should a stricter method be applied to diagnosing individuals with ADHD?
3. The data shows that nonmedical use of ADHD stimulant medication is increasing. What are preventative measures that can be taken to decrease nonmedical use? Should there be greater restrictions on the administration of stimulant medications?
4. There is a definite gender difference in the prevalence of ADHD. Why do you think ADHD is more prevalent among males than females?
5. There is not a substantial body of research on the risk factors for ADHD. Aside from gender, what other possible risk factors for ADHD should be studied?

2

ALCOHOL CONSUMPTION

INTRODUCTION

What Is Alcohol?

Alcohol is a flammable, intoxicating substance found in wine, beer, and other drinks. It is also in some medical liquids, like rubbing alcohol. Alcohol is called a depressant because it slows reaction time, vital signs, digestion, and one's ability to think clearly and make rational decisions.

There are a number of different types of alcoholic beverages. Beer is a common and a cheap alcoholic drink, made from barley, and is known for having a relatively low alcohol content. Wine is a more formal drink, made from grapes, and can be very expensive depending on the year, or "vintage." Hard alcohol, like tequila, whiskey, and vodka, is a distilled, meaning it is concentrated, and has a higher proof (alcohol content) than other drinks. The average serving of hard alcohol is 40–50% alcohol, whereas beer is only 3–5%.

Alcohol Consumption as a Health Issue

There are a number of ways alcohol consumption can become a health issue. One of these is binge drinking, which is most commonly seen in college parties. Binge drinking is said to occur when a person takes a large number of drinks in a short time, resulting in a high blood alcohol concentration (BAC), loss of judgment, and various physical impairments. In some cases, passing out and vomiting are possible. Binge drinking among young adults often occurs as part of social drinking activities, such as doing shots or playing drinking games, such as beer pong.

Excessive consumption of alcohol can also result in alcohol poisoning. The general signs of alcohol poisoning are:

- Confusion
- Slurred speech
- Slowed breathing
- Slowed pulse
- Seizures
- Irregular breathing (often stopping and starting)
- Low body temperature
- Passing out (and unable to be woken up)
- Blue or pale skin

Regular consumption of alcohol over a period of time can also result in alcoholism. Alcoholism is when a person becomes physically or mentally dependent on alcohol, causing him or her to drink more at one time as well as more frequently, interfering with personal relationships, work, and other factors. Alcoholics are also more likely to drink in risky situations, like when driving, and tend to wind up in legal trouble. Some indicators of alcoholism are:

- After drinking, the person cannot remember events from during or before they began (blacking out)
- The person needs to drink more to get the same effect (increased tolerance)
- He or she keeps drinking despite it causing or worsening health issues, like liver disease
- The person gives up other activities to drink
- A significant amount of time is dedicated to drinking and recovering from the ensuing hangovers
- Drinking early in the day
- Drinking for long periods of time
- Often drinking alone
- Unusual weight loss, stomach pains and chronic redness of the face

- Withdrawal symptoms if he or she does not consume alcohol for 4–12 hours

Individuals who regularly consume alcohol and then stop abruptly may face withdrawal symptoms, which can range from uncomfortable to life-threatening. Withdrawal symptoms can include:

- Vomiting
- Sweating
- Shaking
- Anxiety
- Headaches
- Confusion
- Hallucinations
- Seizures
- Death (in rare cases)

DATA AND ANALYSES

Data

Table 2.1 Progressive Effects of Alcohol

Blood alcohol concentration	Changes in feelings and personality	Physical and mental impairments
0.01–0.06	Relaxation Sense of well-being Loss of inhibition Lowered alertness Joyous	Thought Judgment Coordination Concentration
0.06–0.10	Blunted feelings Disinhibition Extroversion Impaired sexual pleasure	Impaired reflexes Reasoning Depth perception Distance acuity Peripheral vision Glare recovery
0.11–0.20	Over-expression Emotional swings Angry or sad Boisterous	Reaction time Gross motor control Staggering Slurred speech
0.21–0.29	Stupor Lose understanding Impaired sensations	Severe motor impairment Loss of consciousness Memory blackout

(Continued)

Table 2.1 Progressive Effects of Alcohol (*Continued*)

Blood alcohol concentration	Changes in feelings and personality	Physical and mental impairments
0.30–0.39	Severe depression Unconsciousness Death possible	Bladder function Breathing Heart rate
≥0.40	Unconsciousness Death	Breathing Heart rate

Source: Alcohol's Effects. Campus Alcohol Abuse Prevention Center, Virginia Tech Division of Student Affairs. Retrieved from: http://www.alcohol.vt.edu/Students/Alcohol_effects/index.html

Analysis

Table 2.1 shows the effects of alcohol as more and more of it is consumed. The first category, .01–.06, shows relatively minor changes, with the most notable being joyousness and a heightened sense of well-being. As we move down the table, the effects get noticeably worse, and even at merely .06 we see an impairment of depth perception, reasoning skills, and self-restraint (inhibition). This is why it is illegal to drive with a BAC over .08.

It is also important to note the more severe side effects of alcohol consumption. Once above a .20 BAC, a person may not understand their surroundings and what is going on around them. People who have become that intoxicated are more likely to fall or stumble into the street, where they might be struck by a passing car. Severe depression and poor judgment may lead to a suicide attempt. People who drink a very high amount of alcohol may have their hearts or breathing stop, endangering their lives.

Data

Table 2.2 Alcohol Content Per Drink Size and Type

Standard drink chart (U.S.)				
Alcohol	Amount (ml)	Amount (fl oz)	Serving size	Alcohol (% by vol.)	Alcohol
80-proof liquor	44	1.5	One shot	40	0.6 US fl oz (18 ml)
Table wine	148	5	One glass	12	0.6 US fl oz (18 ml)
Beer	355	12	One can/bottle	5	0.6 US fl oz (18 ml)

Source: http://www.cdc.gov/alcohol/faqs.htm

Analysis

By showing the three main types of alcohol side by side, Table 2.2 illustrates why it is so easy to become intoxicated when taking shots. Since a shot is less than one-third as much liquid as wine (and an eighth as much as beer), but the same amount of alcohol, the unwary drinker could take several shots before feeling like he or she has drank any significant amount of liquid. Since alcohol needs time to take effect, it is easy for a drinker to think shots aren't having a big effect.

Data

Table 2.3 Binge Drinking Prevalence, Frequency, and Intensity Among Adults, by Sociodemographic Characteristics—Behavioral Risk Factor Surveillance System Combined Landline and Cellular Telephone Developmental Dataset, United States,* 2010

	Prevalence			Frequency[†]			Intensity[§]		
Attribute	No.	Weighted %	(95% CI[¶])	No.	No. of episodes	(95% CI)	No.	No. of drinks	(95% CI)
Total	457,677	17.1	(16.8–17.4)	52,329	4.4	(4.3–4.5)	48,683	7.9	(7.8–8.1)
Sex									
Male	176,911	23.2	(22.6–23.7)	30,511	5.0	(4.8–5.1)	28,192	9.0	(8.8–9.2)
Female	280,766	11.4	(11.1–11.8)	21,818	3.2	(3.1–3.4)	20,491	5.9	(5.8–6.0)
Age group (yrs)									
18–24	18,087	28.2	(26.9–29.5)	4,688	4.2	(4.0–4.5)	4,358	9.3	(8.9–9.7)
25–34	42,767	27.9	(26.9–29.0)	9,900	4.2	(3.9–4.4)	9,290	8.4	(8.1–8.6)
35–44	61,216	19.2	(18.4–19.9)	10,902	4.1	(3.9–4.4)	10,259	7.6	(7.3–8.0)
45–64	187,127	13.3	(12.9–13.6)	21,720	4.7	(4.5–4.9)	20,219	6.8	(6.7–7.0)
≥65	144,645	3.8	(3.5–4.0)	4,925	5.5	(4.8–6.2)	4,403	5.7	(5.5–6.0)
Race/Ethnicity									
White, non-Hispanic	359,123	18.0	(17.7–18.4)	42,258	4.4	(4.3–4.5)	39,514	7.9	(7.7–8.0)
Black, non-Hispanic	36,275	12.7	(11.7–13.6)	2,920	4.7	(4.1–5.3)	2,595	6.8	(6.3–7.4)
Hispanic	31,061	17.9	(16.6–19.1)	3,826	3.8	(3.4–4.2)	3,525	8.4	(7.8–9.0)
Other, non-Hispanic	25,137	15.3	(13.8–16.8)	2,881	4.7	(4.2–5.3)	2,671	8.7	(8.0–9.4)
Education level									
Less than high school diploma	42,359	13.7	(12.8–14.6)	3,574	5.5	(5.0–6.0)	3,177	9.3	(8.7–9.9)
High school diploma	135,634	17.6	(17.0–18.1)	15,111	4.7	(4.5–4.9)	13,864	8.2	(8.0–8.4)

(Continued)

Table 2.3 Binge Drinking Prevalence, Frequency, and Intensity Among
Adults, by Sociodemographic Characteristics—Behavioral Risk Factor
Surveillance System Combined Landline and Cellular Telephone
Developmental Dataset, United States,* 2010 (*Continued*)

	Prevalence				Frequency[†]		Intensity[§]		
Attribute	No.	Weighted %	(95% CI[¶])	No.	No. of episodes	(95% CI)	No.	No. of drinks	(95% CI)
Education level Some college	123,093	19.0	(18.4–19.6)	14,795	4.1	(4.0–4.3)	13,767	7.6	(7.5–7.8)
College graduate	155,652	18.2	(17.7–18.7)	18,805	3.4	(3.3–3.5)	17,843	6.9	(6.7–7.0)
Income									
≤$25,000	119,988	16.2	(15.5–16.9)	10,795	5.0	(4.7–5.3)	9,880	8.5	(8.2–8.9)
$25,000–$49,999	108,542	17.9	(17.2–18.5)	12,316	4.2	(4.0–4.4)	11,446	7.9	(7.6–8.1)
$50,000–$74,999	62,539	18.9	(18.1–19.7)	8,484	4.4	(4.1–4.7)	8,058	7.9	(7.6–8.2)
≥$75,000	105,280	20.2	(19.7–20.8)	16,665	3.7	(3.6–3.9)	15,849	7.2	(7.0–7.3)

*Respondents were from 48 states (excluding South Dakota and Tennessee) and the District of Columbia.
[†]Binge drinkers only; average number of binge-drinking episodes per month.
[§]Average largest number of drinks consumed by binge drinkers on any occasion in the past month.
[¶]CI = confidence interval.

Source: http://www.cdc.gov/mmwr/preview/mmwrhtml/mm6101a4.htm?s_cid=mm6101a4_w#tab1

Analysis

One of the most serious issues associated with alcohol consumption is binge drinking. Table 2.3 presents data on the prevalence, frequency and intensity if binge drinking. Approximately 38 million
people (or 1 in 6 of the total population) binge drink. On average,
those who binge drink do so approximately four times per month.
The data shows that the prevalence and intensity of binge drinking
was highest among persons aged 18–34 years. This is not entirely
surprising since heavy drinking can be a pass time for some college students and young adults. However, the table also shows that
the frequency of binge drinking was highest among binge drinkers aged 65 years or older. Socioeconomic status also appears to be
a factor in binge drinking. Binge drinking prevalence was highest
among those with annual household incomes of more than $75,000.
However, binge drinkers with household incomes of less than
$25,000 had the highest frequency and intensity of binge drinking.

DISCUSSION QUESTIONS

1. Alcohol consumption is more popular among young adults
   (21–30) than in other age groups. Why do you think this is?

2. The side effects from overindulging in alcohol can be debilitating and severe, yet thousands drink to excess every year. Should this be allowed, or should something be done to discourage people from drinking that much? If so, what can be done?
3. Do you believe enough is done to educate young people about the dangers of overconsumption of alcohol? Why or why not?
4. Alcoholism is classified as a mental disability, but some feel that drinking is a choice, not an illness. What do you think, and why?

3

ALLERGIES

INTRODUCTION

Understanding Food and Environmental Allergies

Allergies, also known as hypersensitivities, are the immune system's abnormal reaction to a stimulus that does not normally pose a negative affect on people. When the immune system detects the presence of an allergen, antibodies called Immunoglobulin E (IgE) are produced. These antibodies then signal cells to release certain chemicals that cause allergic reactions.

The amount of IgE antibodies in one's body determines the amount of allergens that they will react to. People tend to be allergic to more than one substance or allergen. Allergies are typically divided in to three categories: food allergies, skin allergies, and respiratory allergies. Common substances that produce hypersensitive reactions include food, pollen, dust, mold, pet dander, and insect stings. Cow's milk, eggs, peanuts, wheat, soy, fish, shellfish, and tree nuts account for over 90% of food allergic reactions.

Symptoms

Various symptoms can arise from allergies, at all different severity levels. Additionally, the symptoms can appear in various body locations; however, the most common are the nose, lungs, throat, sinuses, ears, lining of the stomach, or on the skin. The most common conditions and symptoms are:

- Allergic rhinitis/hay fever: Runny nose, sneezing, and itchy, swollen eyes; most commonly caused by environmental allergens such as pollen, dust, mold, or pets
- Allergic conjunctivitis: Red, itchy, swollen eyes; most commonly caused by environmental allergens such as pollen, dust, mold, or pets
- Atopic dermatitis/eczema: Red, itchy, peeling skin; most commonly caused by allergen exposure to the skin
- Urticaria/hives: Itchy, red bumps on the skin; most commonly caused by food or medication allergens
- Asthma: Coughing, shortness of breath, tightening of the chest; most commonly caused by inhaling environmental allergens such as dust or smoke
- Anaphylaxis: Red, itchy rash, tingling of the mouth, light-headedness, anxiety, shortness of breath, vomiting, throat tightness; most commonly caused by food, medications, insect stings, and latex

Diagnosis

Allergists will often complete a physical exam and examine family history when diagnosing for allergies. If allergies are suspected, certain tests can be administered to determine specific allergens.

Allergy skin tests expose the skin to suspected allergens to determine whether there is an allergic reaction that follows. Allergy skin tests can be used for people of all ages; however, allergists should not administer the test if the individual has ever had a case of anaphylaxis, they are taking medications that could interfere with the results such as antihistamines or antidepressants, they have a widespread skin reaction, or they have other skin conditions that interfere with the results. Allergy skin tests are most commonly used to diagnose environmental allergens such as pollen, dust, or pet dander. When undergoing this test, individuals should be aware of a common side effect that presents as swollen, red, itchy bumps on the skin. These bumps normally subside within a few hours after testing.

Allergen-specific IgE antibody tests are blood tests used to diagnose allergies to specific substances. The test will be administered when there are recurrent symptoms, whether they be acute or chronic. The test does not have an affect on the individual; therefore, it can be used as an alternative to allergy skin tests. Additionally, the test can be used to monitor immunotherapy, allergy shots, or to test whether a child has outgrown an allergy.

Additional tests that may be administered are the skin prick test, which tests for allergic reactions to over 40 allergens at once; the skin injection test, which injects a small amount of the allergen in to the skin to observe for allergic reactions; or the patch test, which detects delayed allergic reactions by applying 20–30 allergens to a patch and then placing the patch on an individual's skin.

Risk Factors

It is currently unknown why some substances pose as allergens to certain people. The biggest risk factors for allergic conditions are:

- Family history
- Young age
- Pre-existence of asthma or another allergic condition

Treatment

There is currently no cure for allergies, yet individuals can lead a healthy, normal life with treatment. Once an individual's allergens are identified, allergy shots can be administered, also known as immunotherapy. Additional treatment methods include avoiding allergens, taking allergy medications such as corticosteroids or antihistamines to reduce symptoms, and the administering of emergency epinephrine to prevent anaphylaxis during severe reactions.

DATA AND ANALYSES

Data

Table 3.1 Percentage of Children Aged 0–17 Years with a Reported Allergic Condition, by Age Group: United States, Average Annual 2009–2011

Type of allergy	Percentage of age group 0–4 years	Percentage of age group 5–9 years	Percentage of age group 10–17 years
Food allergy	5%	5.1%	5%
Skin allergy	14.2%	13.1%	10.9%
Respiratory allergy	10.8%	17.4%	20.8%

Source: Akinbami, L.J., Howie, L.D., & Jackson K.D. 2013. "Trends in allergic conditions among children: United States, 1997–2011." National Center for Health Statistics. Retrieved from: http://www.cdc.gov/nchs/data/databriefs/db121.pdf

Analysis

Allergic conditions are some of the most common medical conditions among children in the United States. Between 1997 and 2011, the prevalence of food allergies and skin allergies increased among children aged 0–17 years old. Respiratory allergies remained relatively the same; however, they consistently made up for the most allergies among children during this period.

Table 3.2 breaks this information into age groups, finding that food allergy prevalence was similar among all age groups, affecting about 5% of children. Skin allergies decreased with age, affecting 14.2% of children aged 0–4 and only 10.9% of children aged 10–17. Respiratory allergies increased with age, doubling from affecting 10.8% of children aged 0–4 to 20.8% of children aged 10–17.

By examining the prevalence of allergic conditions in children, allergists will be able to gain a better understanding of what causes allergic conditions and can employ treatment methods to improve quality of life.

Data

Table 3.2 Average Number of Hospital Discharges Per Year Among Children Under Age 18 Years with Any Diagnosis Related to Food Allergy: United States, 1998–2006

Years	Average number of discharges per year
1998–2000	2,615
2001–2003	4,135
2004–2006	9,537

Source: Branum, A.M. & Lukacs, S.L. 2008. "Food allergy among U.S. children: Trends in prevalence and hospitalizations." National Center for Health Statistics. Retrieved from: http://www.cdc.gov/nchs/data/databriefs/db10.htm

Analysis

From 1997 to 2007, the prevalence of food allergies among children under 18 years old increased 18%, resulting in an estimated three million children who suffer from food allergies. Children with food allergies are two to four times more likely to have other allergic conditions such as asthma, which leads to an increased risk of anaphylaxis and hospitalization or death.

Table 3.2 represents the increase in hospitalizations due to food allergies from 1998 to 2006. From 2004 to 2006, there 9,537 hospitalizations of children aged 0–17 years, more than three times the amount between 1998 and 2000.

The increase in hospitalizations may be related to increased awareness, reporting, or use of medical diagnostic codes for food allergies, yet it also could simply represent an increase in the number of children experiencing food allergic reactions. Further research on the subject can examine the cause of food allergic reactions and the establishment of preventative measures to save children from needing hospitalization.

DISCUSSION QUESTIONS

1. Why are respiratory allergies the most common in children? Why have the incidences of respiratory allergies not increased over the years like food allergies and skin allergies?
2. What factors cause an increase or decrease in reported allergies? Why do respiratory allergies increase with age, while skin allergies decrease and food allergies remain the same?
3. How do food allergy hospitalizations compare to respiratory and skin allergy hospitalizations?
4. What is the link between different types of allergies? Why do children with food allergies tend to present with other allergic conditions as well?
5. How can hospitalization be prevented in children with food allergies? What treatment methods are currently being employed for food allergies and are they proving to be effective?

4

ALZHEIMER'S DISEASE

INTRODUCTION

Understanding Alzheimer's Disease

The brain controls all of the processes of the human body. When the brain experiences microscopic changes in the tissues that facilitate learning, memorizing, and moving, this important organ loses its ability to provide the body with the means necessary to carry out daily activities. Alzheimer's disease, a progressive and irreversible condition of which the cause or causes are still unknown, is just one of the diseases that involve these kinds of toxic, microscopic changes. Clumps and tangled fibers form in the brain and inhibit normal behavior and functioning, eventually causing dementia and rendering a person unable to move or communicate.

Symptoms

Memory problems are one of the earliest indicators of Alzheimer's disease. However, as the disease progresses into its mild, moderate, and severe stages, several other symptoms develop around the degenerating cognitive faculties that distinguish them from the simple signs of old age. People who have reached the mild stage of

Alzheimer's disease, which is typically the stage when doctors can provide a diagnosis, usually exhibit the following symptoms:

- Easily getting lost
- Difficulty completing financial tasks, like handling money or paying bills
- Difficulty repeating questions or statements
- Taking a longer time to complete normal tasks
- Easily losing things
- Poor judgment
- Mood swings
- Personality changes

When a person transitions from the mild stage to the moderate stage of Alzheimer's disease, a larger portion of their brain has already been affected. As a result, moderate Alzheimer's disease patients may exhibit any of the following symptoms:

- Increased memory loss
- Increased confusion
- Difficulty recognizing loved ones
- Difficulty learning new things
- Difficulty carrying out multiple-step tasks
- Hallucinations
- Delusions
- Paranoia
- Impulsive behavior

The severe stage of Alzheimer's disease features the most severe symptoms of the condition. During this time, patients are mostly bedridden and completely dependent on their caregivers. Symptoms of the severe stage of Alzheimer's disease include:

- Total inability to communicate
- Weight loss
- Seizures
- Skin infections
- Difficulty swallowing
- Repeating the same word or sound
- Grunting and groaning
- Rocking back and forth
- Incontinence

Risk Factors

Although researchers cannot pinpoint the exact cause of Alzheimer's disease, most of them do agree that there are three main risk factors that play an important part in the development and diagnosis of the condition. These risk factors revolve around age, family history, and genetics.

It is not impossible for young people to have Alzheimer's disease. However, once a person reaches 65 years of age, the risk of getting Alzheimer's disease doubles every five years. When he or she is 85 years old, this risk jumps to 50%.

Also, if a person's parent, sibling, or child has Alzheimer's disease, he or she is more likely to develop it as well. This family history risk factor is linked directly to the genetics risk factor, as genes passed down from generation to generation can significantly impact the likelihood of contracting Alzheimer's disease. Deterministic genes, which directly cause a disease, and risk genes, which increase the likelihood of a disease but do not guarantee the development of it, have both been identified as categories of genes linked to Alzheimer's disease.

Treatment

Although scientists continue to conduct their research on Alzheimer's disease, no definitive cure has been identified for this elusive medical condition. Currently, there are no drugs that completely stop or reverse cell damage caused by Alzheimer's disease, but there are medications that have the ability to subdue certain symptoms of the disease and improve the overall quality of life for a patient struggling through the early to moderate stages, as well as the moderate to severe stages.

Most recently, the United States Food and Drug Administration has approved medications that involve cholinesterase inhibitors, which strengthen nerve communication by preventing important acetylcholine messengers in the body from disintegrating, and memantine, which improves memory and attention by taking control of glutamate messengers. Both cholinesterase inhibitors and memantine medications mask or delay the worsening of symptoms, but they are only temporary fixes.

When prescribed medications do not yield desired results, some patients opt for alternative treatments in the form of herbal remedies or dietary supplements. These can range from coenzyme Q10 antioxidants to coral calcium supplements, and even to extracts of moss or gingko biloba trees. In most cases, the effectiveness and safety of these alternative treatments are not known. Clinical trials have uncovered that some of these alternative treatments simply act as placebos for people with Alzheimer's disease who decide to take them.

Regardless of whether a patient chooses to be treated with pre-scribed medications or alternative methods, he or she usually requires full-time care to administer these treatments and help with normal daily activities such as eating and getting dressed. Alzheim-er's disease patients typically rely on nursing homes, hospices, and hospitals when loved ones or other caregivers are no longer able to provide the proper support.

DATA AND ANALYSES

Data

Table 4.1 Alzheimer's Disease Death Rates in the United States by Age, Age-adjusted, 2000 and 2010

	2000	2010
65–74 years old	18.7	19.8
75–84 years old	139.6	184.5
85 years and older	667.1	987.1
Total data	825.4	1,191.4

Note: Rates are per 10,000 population and age-adjusted.

Source: NCHS Data Brief, Number 116, March 2013, Mortality from Alzheimer's Disease in the United States: Data for 2000 and 2010. Retrieved from: http://www.cdc.gov/nchs/data/databriefs/db116.htm

Analysis

Data collected and compiled by the Centers for Disease Control and Prevention from the National Vital Statistics System shows that people in the United States seem to have a greater risk of dying from Alzheimer's disease as they grow older. In both 2000 and 2010, people 85 years and older were more likely to die from Alzheimer's disease than younger age groups. In fact, in 2010 alone this age range was more than 50 times more likely to die than people aged 65–74, and five times more likely than people aged 75–84.

However, the Table 4.1 does not only confirm that the risk of dying from Alzheimer's disease in the United States increases dramatically with age. It also provides evidence to support that the risk of dying from the condition has increased from 2000 to 2010 for all age groups. For people aged 65–74, the death rate increased 6% starting at 18.7 in 2000 and ending the decade at 19.8 in 2010. For people aged 75–84, the death rate jumped 32% from 139.6 in 2000 to 184.5 in 2010. For people aged 85 and over, there was a 48% increase from 667.1 in 2000 to 987.1 in 2010. Overall, the death rate for these three age groups spiked significantly, going from 825.4 in 2000 to 1,191.4 in 2010.

Data

Table 4.2 Alzheimer's Disease Death Rates in the United States by State, Age-adjusted, 2010

Death rate range	States
10.5 to 19.9	Connecticut, District of Columbia, Florida, Hawaii, Maryland, Nevada, New Jersey, New Mexico, New York, Utah
20.0 to 29.9	Alaska, Arkansas, Delaware, Georgia, Idaho, Illinois, Indiana, Kansas, Maine, Massachusetts, Michigan, Minnesota, Missouri, Montana, Nebraska, New Hampshire, Ohio, Oklahoma, Oregon, Pennsylvania, Rhode Island, Texas, Virginia, West Virginia, Wisconsin, Wyoming
30.0 to 39.9	Alabama, Arizona, California, Colorado, Iowa, Kentucky, Louisiana, Mississippi, North Carolina, North Dakota, South Carolina, South Dakota, Tennessee, Vermont
40 and over	Washington

Note: Rates are age-adjusted.

Source: NCHS Data Brief, Number 116, March 2013, Mortality from Alzheimer's Disease in the United States: Data for 2000 and 2010. Retrieved from: http://www.cdc.gov/nchs/data/databriefs/db116.htm

Analysis

In the United States, Alzheimer's disease death rates vary from state to state. Although each state death rate in the country fits into a ranged category in Table 4.2, there seems to be no consistent geographic pattern across the states.

In general, the lowest incidence of deaths caused by Alzheimer's disease were found in Connecticut, District of Columbia, Florida, Hawaii, Maryland, Nevada, New Jersey, New Mexico, New York, and Utah. The state with the highest death rate was Washington. The remaining 40 states fell in the 20.0–39.9 death rate range. There are many reasons why death rates for Alzheimer's may vary from state to state. Further research into these geographic differences may help scientists to better understand the progression of the disease and the efficacy of currently available treatments.

DISCUSSION QUESTIONS

1. Although researchers have not yet pinpointed a definitive cause for Alzheimer's disease, they continue to study the condition and conduct experiments to better understand it. Can you think of a few possible tests researchers would be able to conduct on brain cells to establish a cure more quickly?
2. Table 4.1 shows that the risk of patients dying from Alzheimer's disease has actually increased from 2000 to 2010. What are some possible reasons for the dramatic increase in death rate during this decade?
3. The three main risk factors of Alzheimer's, which include age, family history, and genetics, are largely unpreventable. What do you think are some factors connected to the condition that patients have the ability to control or influence?
4. Memory loss is a problem associated with old age, but people who have difficulty remembering things as they age do not necessarily have Alzheimer's disease. How might doctors providing a diagnosis distinguish between old age and Alzheimer's disease?
5. The Centers for Disease Control and Prevention stresses that Alzheimer's disease is not a normal part of aging. If age is one of the greatest risk factors of the condition, how can this be?

5

ANEMIA

INTRODUCTION

Understanding Anemia

Hemoglobin is an iron-rich protein constituent of red blood cells that enables oxygen to be carried from the lungs throughout the body, and to carry carbon dioxide out of the body through the lungs. With abnormal or low counts of red blood cells or hemoglobin, the cells in the body will lack oxygen, leading to a condition known as anemia. Most red blood cells and hemoglobin are produced regularly in bone marrow. To support this production, iron, vitamin B_{12}, folate, and other nutrients are necessary.

As the most common blood condition in the United States, anemia affects an estimated 3.5 million Americans. There are over 400 different types of anemia, varying in causes and treatment. The three main causes of anemia include:

- Anemia caused by blood loss: Chronic blood loss occurs slowly over a long period of time and often goes undetected. Related causes include gastrointestinal conditions, use of nonsteroidal anti-inflammatory drugs, menstruation, and childbirth. Iron deficiency anemia is the most common condition.

- Anemia caused by decreased or abnormal red blood cell production: A lack of minerals and vitamins may cause decreased or abnormal red blood cell production. Associated conditions include sickle cell anemia, vitamin deficiency, and bone marrow and other chronic diseases.
- Anemia caused by the destruction of red blood cells: Weak red blood cells may rupture, causing hemolytic anemia. Related causes include hereditary conditions, lifestyle stressors, toxins from other diseases, tumors, hypertension, and other disorders.

Symptoms

Symptoms of anemia tend to increase as the condition worsens. Severity and types of symptoms vary depending on the cause of the disease, yet all symptoms are produced because the heart must work harder to pump oxygen-rich blood throughout the body. Fatigue is the most common symptom; however, others include:

- Pale skin
- Fast or irregular heartbeats
- Shortness of breath
- Chest pain
- Dizziness
- Cognitive problems
- Cold hands and feet
- Headaches

Diagnosis

Since anemic conditions are often mild at the start, they may go undetected. It is important to contact a doctor if unexplained feelings of fatigue arise. Tests used to diagnose anemia include:

- Physical exams: A doctor may listen to an individual's heart for rapid or irregular beating, as well as their lungs for rapid or uneven breathing. They also may feel the size of the liver and the spleen.
- Complete blood count (CBC): The number of blood cells in a sample of blood is counted to determine the level of red blood cells and hemoglobin. Normal red blood cell counts for adults vary, but are generally between 38.8 and 50% for males and 34.9 and 44.5% for women. Normal hemoglobin counts for

adults are generally 13.5–17.5 grams per deciliter for males and 12–15.5 grams per deciliter for females. Also, CBC checks the mean corpuscular volume, which measures average size of red blood cells.

- Other tests may be administered, as an unusual size, shape or color of red blood cells may help determine what type of anemia is present.
  - Hemoglobin electrophoresis: Examines the type of hemoglobin in the blood
  - Reticulocyte count: Measures the number of young red blood cells to determine the production rate of the bone marrow
  - Serum iron, serum ferritin, transferrin level, and total iron-binding capacity tests: Measure iron levels

Risk Factors

As anemia is the most common type of blood disorder, there are various risk factors that individuals should be aware of, including:

- Nutrition: Diets that lack iron, vitamin B_{12}, and folate increase risks of developing anemia.
- Intestinal disorders: These disorders affect the absorption of nutrients in the small intestine, which leads to an increased risk of anemia.
- Menstruation: Young women who have begun menstruation are at higher risk of developing anemia, due to the loss of red blood cells that occurs.
- Pregnancy: During the first six months of pregnancy, the fluid portion of a woman's blood increases faster than the number of red blood cells diluting the blood, leading to a depletion of iron stores and risk of iron-deficiency anemia.
- Newborns and infants: Young children are at risk if they are born too early or are not fed with formula or milk that is fortified with iron. Many children drink cow's milk, which is low in iron.
- Chronic conditions: Anemia of chronic disease occurs when chronic conditions cause a shortage of red blood cells and deplete the body of iron.
- Family history: Certain types of anemia are hereditary, so infants with a family history of anemic conditions are at risk of developing anemia from the time of birth.
- Other: Certain blood disorders and autoimmune diseases, alcoholism, toxic chemicals, and some medications also lead to an increased risk of anemia.

Treatment

Left untreated, anemia can cause severe fatigue, heart problems, and even death; therefore, it is important to seek treatment as soon as possible. Treatment options vary based on the cause of the anemia. The main goal of treatment is to increase the amount of oxygen that the blood can carry by raising the red blood cell and hemoglobin levels, or to treat the underlying condition causing anemia.

- Anemia caused by blood loss: Changes in diet and taking iron supplements for iron deficiency anemia can be used as treatment. Iron can be easily absorbed from eating meats, but also from spinach and dark green leafy vegetables, tofu, beans, and lentils, etc.
- Anemia caused by decreased or abnormal red blood cell production: Folic acid and vitamin C supplements or vitamin B_{12} injections are common treatments for vitamin-deficiency anemia. For anemia of chronic disease, chemotherapy, bone marrow transplants, or other surgery may be necessary.
- Anemia caused by the destruction of red blood cells: Related infections are treated by taking drugs that suppress the immune system that may be attacking red blood cells. In hemolytic anemia cases, blood transfusions or plasmapheresis may be necessary. Sickle cell anemia and other conditions may require bone marrow transplants or other surgeries.

DATA AND ANALYSES

Data

Table 5.1 Global Anemia Prevalence and Number of Individuals Affected

Population group	Age range	Prevalence of anemia (Percent)	Population affected (Number in millions)
Preschool-age children	0–4.99	47.4	293
School-age children	5–14.99	25.4	305
Pregnant women	No age range	41.8	56
Non-pregnant women	15–50	30.2	468
Men	15–60	12.7	260
Elderly	Older than 60	23.9	164
Total population	All ages	24.8	1620

Source: Benoist, B., Cogswell, M., Egli, I., & McLean, E. 2008. "Worldwide prevalence of anaemia: 1993–2005." World Health Organization. Retrieved from: http://whqlibdoc.who.int/publications/2008/9789241596657_eng.pdf?ua=1

Analysis

As Table 5.1 presents, anemia affects approximately 1.62 billion people worldwide, which amounts to an estimate of 25% of the world's population. As a major contributing factor to global diseases, population groups across the globe were categorized by age to study the trends of anemia throughout the life cycle.

Based on the specific population groups, preschool-age children presented the greatest prevalence of anemia, followed by pregnant and nonpregnant women. However, based on the amount of individuals in each population group, anemia affects nonpregnant women the most, followed by school-age and preschool-age children. Since there is a smaller population of pregnant women, they present the lowest number of individuals affected even though this number is a high percentage of the pregnant female population. Additionally, males produced the lowest prevalence and affected rates of anemia. While the elderly are at a high risk for anemia, the global perspective of this data shows that addressing anemia prevalence in young children is critical. In underdeveloped countries, the disease may prevent many individuals from aging, resulting in the smaller prevalence of anemia in the world's elderly population.

The presented data complies with the risk factors for anemia, showing that women and children are most susceptible to the disease. Worldwide, anemia affects about a quarter of the population, displaying the severity of its prevalence. Further research needs to be done to determine which types of anemia account for the data presented. By examining the types of anemia that are present, further preventative and treatment measures can be determined.

Data

Table 5.2 Anemia-related Deaths by Age in the United States, 2010

Age	Number of deaths caused by anemia
Under 1 year	15
1 to 4 years	29
5 to 14 years	26
15 to 24 years	109
25 to 34 years	142
35 to 44 years	178
45 to 54 years	264
55 to 64 years	369

(Continued)

Table 5.2 Anemia-related Deaths by Age in the United States, 2010 (*Continued*)

Age	Number of deaths caused by anemia
65 to 74 years	524
75 to 84 years	1,091
85 years and over	2,104
Age not stated	1
Total	4,852

Source: Kochanek, K.D., Murphy, S.L., & Xu, J. 2010. "Deaths: Final data for 2010. National vital statistics report." Retrieved from: http://www.cdc.gov/nchs/fastats/anemia.htm

Analysis

Table 5.2 more closely examines the number of individuals affected by anemia categorized by age-group populations. Specifically, the data table focuses on solely individuals from the United States. Ultimately 4,852 deaths were attributed to anemia during 2010. To compare, the leading cause of death in the United States, heart disease, accounted for 780,213 deaths in 2010. While the number of deaths related to anemia may not appear as severe as heart disease or other causes, there is a trend related to age.

The table shows that there is a direct relationship between age and anemia prevalence, specifically that anemia prevalence increases with age. As age progresses, the number of anemia-related deaths increases almost twofold. There were 2,104 anemia-related deaths in those 85 years and older, the highest out of all age-group populations. While this data may seem to contradict the global prevalences of anemia based on age-group populations, it is important to consider the living conditions of the United States. As a developed country, the United States has the ability to provide nourishment for young children, eliminating a major amount of anemia-related deaths in the younger age groups. Additionally, the resources and medicine required to extend the lifespan are available in the United States, allowing more people to reach the ages of 85 and older. In other less developed countries around the world, the ability to sustain life is shortened, which leads to the smaller affects on the elderly.

In the United States, the relationship between age and anemia-related deaths is supported by major risk factors. The elderly are at greater risk of developing chronic diseases and nutritional deficiencies, which leads to the presence of anemia. By further examining the relationship between anemia development and chronic diseases among the elderly, the number of anemia-related deaths can try to be contained. Additionally, the table shows the importance of providing health care from a young age, as other countries that do not have the same abilities as the United States contribute to a large population of anemia-related deaths in young individuals.

DISCUSSION QUESTIONS

1. What are the anemia-related mortality rates of the worldwide population groups? Which age-group suffers greater from a global perspective?
2. What is the breakdown of anemia prevalence by country? How do the economic and living conditions of these countries relate to anemia prevalence?
3. How can other countries attack the issue of anemia in young age-group populations? Can the United States provide information and resources to prevent anemia in these age groups?
4. How can the United States decrease the number of anemia-related deaths in the elderly?
5. What are the greatest causes of anemia in the elderly? Which of these causes is related to the highest number of anemia-related deaths?

6

ARTHRITIS

INTRODUCTION

Understanding Arthritis

The term arthritis does not refer to a single ailment. Rather, the term refers to approximately 120 different diseases, all of which can affect the joints, muscles, and other soft tissues. Of all of the disorders that fall under the arthritis umbrella, the most common forms are:

Osteoarthritis: Osteoarthritis, the most common type of arthritis, involves destruction of the cartilage on the ends of the bones. Over time, damage to one's cartilage can lead to bone grinding directly on bone, which, in turn, can lead to pain and restricted movement.

Fibromyalgia: Fibromyalgia causes pain and stiffness in the tissues that support and move the bones and joints. Individuals suffering from fibromyalgia may also suffer from significant fatigue, sleep disturbances, and difficulty concentrating.

Rheumatoid arthritis: Rheumatoid arthritis is an autoimmune disease that primarily affects the synovial membrane, the lining of the joint capsule. Eventually, the disease can destroy cartilage and bone within the joint. In addition to joint swelling, individuals with rheumatoid arthritis may also experience fevers, fatigue, and a general malaise.

Other forms of arthritis which are less common include: Other types of arthritis include bursitis, tendinitis, gout, systemic lupus erythematosus, juvenile arthritis, scleroderma, ankylosing spondylitis, psoriatic arthritis infectious arthritis, and carpal tunnel syndrome.

Risk Factors for Arthritis

Arthritis can affect people of all ages, including children. There are a number of risks factors for arthritis, including:

- Being 45 years of age and older
- Having a family history of arthritis
- Being African American
- Being obese
- Having sustained injuries to one's joints
- Having an infections, such as Lyme disease
- Being employed in certain occupations that require frequent repetitive joint activities (e.g., kneeling or stooping)

Symptoms of Arthritis

The most common symptoms of arthritis are pain, swelling, and stiffness in joints. Individuals suffering from arthritis may also have difficulty moving the joint normally or suffer from a decreased range of motion in the affected joint(s). In certain forms of arthritis, individuals may experience symptoms outside of the joints. For example, individuals with rheumatoid arthritis may suffer from general malaise, fever, fatigue, weight loss, and swollen lymph glands.

Diagnosing Arthritis

There is no single test for arthritis. Rather, a diagnosis of the disease is based on the pattern of symptoms one experiences, as well as one's medical history, family history, physical examination, and the results of medical tests, including X-rays, computerized tomography (CT) scans, magnetic resonance imaging (MRI), and ultrasounds. In certain cases, physicians may also inspect the joint for damage in your joint by inserting an arthroscope (a small, flexible tube) through an incision near your joint.

Treating Arthritis

There is no cure for arthritis. However, with appropriate disease management, individuals can live healthy lives. Various drug therapies can help to improve joint health and reduce pain. Key to disease management are self-management skills, such as exercise. Exercise plays an important role in preserving joint mobility and for maintaining flexibility. Physical activity can also help afflicted individuals to lose weight, which, in turn, will ease the burden on the joints.

Drug therapy also plays an important role in managing the pain of arthritis and, in some cases, controlling the symptoms of the disease. Depending on the extent of the disease, the following drugs may be prescribed to a person suffering from arthritis.

Corticosteroids: Corticosteroids reduces inflammation and suppresses the immune system. Drugs in this class can be injected directly into the affected joint or may be taken orally. Examples of corticosteroids include prednisone and cortisone.

Nonsteroidal anti-inflammatory drugs (NSAIDs): NSAIDs reduce both pain and inflammation. Typically, NSAIDS may be taken orally but some NSAIDs are applied topically as creams or gels, which can be rubbed on joints. Examples of NSAIDs include ibuprofen and naproxen.

Analgesics: Analgesics reduce pain but have no effect on inflammation. As such, they do not treat the disease but can help individuals who are suffering from painful arthritis symptoms. Examples of analgesics include acetaminophen, tramadol, and narcotics containing oxycodone or hydrocodone.

Disease-modifying antirheumatic drugs (DMARDs): DMARDs actually treat arthritis. They can slow or stop an affected person's immune system from attacking their joints. These drugs are often used to treat rheumatoid arthritis. Examples of DMARDs include methotrexate and hydroxychloroquine.

Biologics: Biologic response modifiers or "biologics" are genetically engineered drugs that target various protein molecules that are involved in the immune response. They are typically used in conjunction with DMARDs. Examples of biologics include etanercept and infliximab.

DATA AND ANALYSES

Data

Table 6.1 Causes of Disability Among U.S. Adults

Cause of disability	Number (in millions) among 47.5 million U.S. adults reporting a disability
Arthritis or rheumatism	**8.6**
Spine or back problems	7.6
Heart trouble	3.0
Lung or respiratory problems	2.2
Mental or emotional problems	2.2
Diabetes	2.0
Deafness or hearing impairment	1.9
Stiffness or deformities of the limbs/ extremities	1.6
Blindness or vision problems	1.5
Stroke	1.1

Source: http://www.cdc.gov/arthritis/data_statistics/national_nhis_text.htm#6

Analysis

As Table 6.1 shows, arthritis is the leading cause of disability among adults in the United States. As discussed above in connection with a review of the risk factors of arthritis,

- Being 45 years of age and older
- Having a family history of arthritis
- Being African American
- Being obese
- Having sustained injuries to one's joints
- Having an infections, such as Lyme disease
- Being employed in certain occupations that require frequent repetitive joint activities (e.g., kneeling or stooping)

For certain forms of arthritis, such as rheumatoid arthritis, there is not anything that one can do to prevent the development of the disorder. However, most cases of arthritis develop as a result of wear and tear on the joint over time. Taking care of one's joints by maintaining a healthy weight and avoiding repetitive joint motions may help to reduce the risks of developing arthritis.

Data

Table 6.2 Projected Prevalence of Doctor-Diagnosed Arthritis, U.S. Adults Aged 18+ years, 2005–2030

Year	Estimated number of adults with doctor-diagnosed arthritis (in 1,000s)		
	Men	Women	Total
2005	18,480	29,358	47,838
2010	20,178	31,701	51,879
2015	21,732	33,993	55,725
2020	23,164	36,244	59,409
2025	24,622	38,587	63,209
2030	26,053	40,915	66,969

Source: http://www.cdc.gov/arthritis/data_statistics/national_nhis_text.htm#6

Analysis

Table 6.2 examines the projected prevalence of doctor-diagnosed arthritis through the year 2030. A review of the table demonstrates a steady increase in the number of diagnosed cases of arthritis. The increase in arthritis is impacting both men and women, at a fairly similar rate of increase.

Data

Table 6.3 Body Mass Index Categories Among Adults With and Without Arthritis in 2002

Body Mass Index category	Arthritis status	
	Doctor-diagnosed arthritis	No arthritis
Underweight/normal	31.2%	43.9%
Overweight	34.0%	35.1%
Obese	34.8%	21.0%

Source: http://www.cdc.gov/arthritis/data_statistics/national_nhis_text.htm

Analysis

Table 6.3 shows that arthritis is more prevalent in those who are overweight or obese than those who are underweight or are of a weight considered normal. Over time, excess weight puts pressure on one's joints and can lead to significant harm to those joints.

Weight management thus has an important role to play in reducing the likelihood that one will suffer from arthritis and, for those that are afflicted by the disease, reducing the severity of the symptoms.

DISCUSSION QUESTIONS

1. According to the data set forth in Table 6.2, the number of cases of arthritis is expected to continue to increase. What can be done to reduce the prevalence of arthritis in the United States?
2. Table 6.3 demonstrates a link between an increased body mass index and a diagnosis of arthritis. Obesity is also the cause of a number of other health problems. What else can our public health system be doing to reduce obesity in order to help protect joint health?
3. Certain activities such as yoga may help to protect joint health and prevent or delay certain forms of arthritis. What else can be done to increase the access that members of the general public has to professionals who can help them to develop a practice in yoga or another form of bodywork?
4. Approximately 60% of patients with untreated infection with Lyme disease may begin to have intermittent bouts of arthritis. For these individuals, arthritis typically presents with severe joint pain and swelling. Lyme disease is transmitted by a bite from an infected tick. Given the severe and often long-lasting consequences of Lyme disease, what more can be done to prevent Lyme disease infections?
5. Table 6.2 demonstrates that the number of diagnosed cases of arthritis is increasing. What are some possible causes for this increase?

7

ASTHMA

INTRODUCTION

Asthma is a relatively common chronic airway disorder characterized by periods of reversible airflow obstruction known as asthma attacks. Airflow may be obstructed by inflammation and airway hyperreactivity (contraction of the small muscles surrounding the airways) in reaction to certain exposures. Exposures include exercise, infection, allergens (e.g., pollen), occupational exposures (e.g., chemicals), and airborne irritants (e.g., environmental tobacco smoke).

Possible Causes and Prevention

While the exact reasons as to why people develop asthma are unclear, there are some theories as to the possible causal factors that may be involved in the development of autism. One cause that is fairly hard to avoid is your genes. If a person's parents tend to suffer from a notable amount of allergies to things like pollen or pet dander (things you breathe in), or if those parents had asthma, then it is more likely that a person will develop asthma to some extent or another later in life.

Respiratory infections during childhood have been linked to asthma, though it is not clear if these infections cause asthma or simply indicate weak airways. However, keeping young children healthy and free of infection may reduce the likelihood of asthma later on.

During early childhood, the immune system is still developing, so exposure to some allergens and infections may contribute to developing asthma. However, another theory states that not being exposed to enough allergens makes the immune system stay weak and react violently later on, so the research here can be conflicting.

Symptoms

The presentation of asthma varies considerably from one individual to another. For some individuals is not more than a minor nuisance that is aggravated by certain environmental stimuli. For other individuals, however, asthma can lead to life-threatening attacks.

The general symptoms of asthma and its warning signs include:

- Frequent cough, especially at night
- Losing your breath easily or shortness of breath
- Feeling very tired or weak when exercising
- Wheezing or coughing after exercise
- Feeling tired, easily upset, grouchy, or moody
- Decreases or changes in lung function as measured on a peak flow meter
- Signs of a cold or allergies (sneezing, runny nose, cough, nasal congestion, sore throat, and headache)
- Trouble sleeping

A number of these symptoms can and do occur independently of asthma however so an examination by a physician will always be necessary to determine whether the symptoms described above are caused by asthma or are the result of something else. Asthma also changes over time. As such, individuals who suspect that they might have asthma or who have been diagnosed with asthma are often advised to track their symptoms over time.

For individuals that do have asthma, attention must be paid to the signs and symptoms of a possible asthma attack. An asthma attack is when your airways become constricted, leading to the inability to breath. Some signs airway obstruction may include:

- Severe wheezing when breathing both in and out
- Coughing that won't stop
- Very rapid breathing

- Chest pain or pressure
- Tightened neck and chest muscles, called retractions
- Difficulty talking
- Feelings of anxiety or panic
- Pale, sweaty face
- Blue lips or fingernails

There are a number of factors that can contribute to the triggering of an asthma attack. Some common triggers include:

- Allergens from dust, animal fur, cockroaches, mold, dust mites, and pollens from trees, grasses, and flowers
- Irritants such as cigarette smoke, air pollution, chemicals, or dust in the workplace, compounds in home décor products, and sprays (such as hairspray)
- Medicines such as aspirin, or other nonsteroidal anti-inflammatory drugs including ibuprofen (Advil, Motrin IB, others) and naproxen (Aleve) and nonselective beta-blockers
- Sulfites and preservatives added to certain foods and drinks
- Viral upper respiratory infections, such as colds
- Physical activity, including exercise (leading to exercise-induced asthma)
- Cold air
- Stress and strong emotions
- Gastroesophageal reflux disease (GERD)

As such, individuals who suffer from asthma would be well advised to take precautions to avoid or at least reduce exposure to the above triggers where possible.

DATA AND ANALYSES

Data

Table 7.1 Asthma Prevalence, by Selected Demographic Characteristics: United States, Average Annual 2008–2010

Category	Percent (standard error)
Total	8.2 (0.1)
Children aged 0–17 years	9.5 (0.2)
Adults aged 18 years and over	7.7 (0.1)

(Continued)

Wellness by the Numbers

Table 7.1 Asthma Prevalence, by Selected Demographic Characteristics: United States, Average Annual 2008–2010 (*Continued*)

Category	Percent (standard error)
Male	7.0 (0.2)
Female	9.2 (0.2)
White	7.7 (0.1)
Black	11.2 (0.3)
American Indian or Alaska Native	9.4 (1.4)
Asian	5.2 (0.4)
Multiple races	14.1 (1.0)
Total Latino	6.5 (0.2)
Puerto Rican	16.1 (1.0)
Mexican	5.4 (0.3)
Less than 100% poverty	11.2 (0.3)
Between 100 to less than 200% poverty	8.7 (0.2)
More than 200%	7.3 (0.1)

Source: Centers for Disease Control, Data Brief 94. Trends in Asthma Prevalence, Health Care Use, and Mortality in the United States, 2001–2010. Retrieved from: http://www.cdc. gov/nchs/data/databriefs/db94_tables.pdf#2

Analysis

Table 7.1 shows very distinct differences in what groups are affected by asthma. For instance, while 8.2% of the total population is affected, only 5.2% of Asian people are affected. However, Puerto Ricans tend to have an astounding 16.2% asthmatic rate. Also interesting is the fact that some children who have it seem to grow out of it, as demonstrated by the higher rate among minors than those over 18. In addition, according to this data, asthma is more prevalent among women than men.

Data

Table 7.2 Asthma Prevalence: United States, 2001–2010

Year	Asthma prevalence (percent/standard error)
2001	7.3
2002	7.2
2003	6.9
2004	7.1
2005	7.7
2006	7.8
2007	7.7

Year	Asthma prevalence (percent/standard error)
2008	7.8
2009	8.2
2010	8.4

Source: Data Brief 94. Trends in Asthma Prevalence, Health Care Use, and Mortality in the United States, 2001–2010. Retrieved from: http://www.cdc.gov/nchs/data/databriefs/db94_tables.pdf#1

Analysis

As Table 7.2 demonstrates, asthma has become more prevalent over the last few years, with these rates spiking upward in 2004–2005 as well as 2008–2009. This indicates a steady decline in lung health among a notable portion of the population, though what portion this might be is unclear.

DISCUSSION QUESTIONS

1. Asthma prevalence increased from 2001 to 2010 and is now at its highest level. What are some possible reasons for this increased prevalence?
2. Why do you think some races might be so prone to asthma while others are not?
3. Some medicine may cause asthma. Do you believe this should be on the label? Should doctors have to say this prior to prescribing the medication? Should people be allowed to sell it at all?
4. Some research suggests that exposure to allergens when young causes asthma, while different research shows it is the *lack* of exposure that causes it. Which do you believe is right? Why?
5. Strong chemicals and tobacco smoke are a few of the airborne irritants that can cause asthma or lead to an attack. Should their use be allowed in public, considering that doing so may inadvertently harm someone?

8

AUTISM

INTRODUCTION

Autism spectrum disorders (ASDs) are a group of developmental disabilities that are characterized by persistent deficits in social communication and social interaction and restricted, repetitive patterns of behavior, interests, or activities. In order to be diagnosed with ASD, symptoms must be present in the early developmental period (typically recognized in the first two years of life) and must cause clinically significant impairment in social, occupational, or other important areas of current functioning. The impact of an ASD can range from mild to significantly disabling, depending on various factors.

There are three different types of ASDs: (1) Autistic disorder (also called "classic" autism and commonly referred to simply as autism); (2) Asperger's syndrome; and (3) pervasive developmental disorder, not otherwise specified (PDD-NOS) (also called "atypical autism"). Significant language delays, social and communication challenges, as well as atypical behaviors and interests characterize autistic disorders. Individuals with Asperger's syndrome usually have some milder symptoms of autistic disorder. While these individuals typically do not suffer from language delays or intellectual disabilities, they might experience social challenges and have unusual behaviors and interests. Individuals who meet some but not all of the diagnostic criteria for autism may be diagnosed with PDD-NOS. Individuals with PDD-NOS typically have fewer and milder symptoms than those with autistic disorder.

ASDs are quite prevalent in the United States and diagnoses continue to increase. Currently, approximately 1 out of 88 children are diagnosed with an ASD. The disorders occur in all socioeconomic, racial, and ethnic groups. It also occurs in both genders but is nearly five times more common about boys than girls, occurring in 1 out of 54 boys and in 1 out of 252 girls.

Indicators and Symptoms

ASDs can be difficult to diagnosis. There are no blood tests or other medical tests to diagnose the disorders. Instead, practitioners examine the behavior and development of the child in order to make a diagnosis. Typically, indicators of autism emerge before a child reaches the age of three. While no particular behavior, or lack of behavior will, in and of itself indicate autism, an individual with autism might:

- Fail to respond to their name by the time he or she reaches 12 months of age
- Not point at objects to show interest by the time he or she reaches 14 months of age
- Not play "pretend" games by the time he or she is 18 months
- Tend to avoid eye contact and want to be alone
- Have trouble understanding other people's feelings or expressing his or her own feelings
- Experience delayed speech and language skills
- Repeat words or phrases over and over
- Give unrelated answers to questions
- Get upset by minor changes
- Have obsessive interests
- Flap their hands, rock their body, or spin in circles
- Have unusual reactions to the way things sound, smell, taste, look, or feel

Treatments and Therapeutic Interventions

Although there continues to be a significant amount of research into ASDs, there is currently no cure for ASDs. Nonetheless, early intervention treatment services can be very effective in improving a child's development. Early intervention services may include therapies designed to help the affected child communicate and interact with others.

Causal Factors

It is currently thought that a number of different factors, including environmental, biologic, and genetic factors, can contribute to making a child more likely to have an ASD. Research suggests that there may be a genetic component in ASDs since children who have a sibling or parent with an ASD are at a higher risk of also having an ASD, and ASDs tend to occur more often in people who have certain genetic or chromosomal conditions, including Down syndrome, fragile X syndrome, and tuberous sclerosis. Certain prenatal factors may also play a role in the development of ASDs. For example, research has shown that when taken during pregnancy, the prescription drugs valproic acid and thalidomide have been linked with a higher risk of ASDs. There have also been suggestions that vaccines and certain infections increase the risk of developing ASDs. However, this remains an issue of considerable controversy.

DATA AND ANALYSES

Data

Table 8.1 Identified Prevalence of Autism Spectrum Disorders

Surveillance year	Birth year	Prevalence per 1,000 children	This is about 1 in X
2000	1992	6.7	1 in 150
2002	1994	6.6	1 in 150
2004	1996	8	1 in 125
2006	1998	11	1 in 110
2008	2000	14	1 in 88

Source: http://www.cdc.gov/ncbddd/autism/data.html

Analysis

Table 8.1 presents data on the prevalence of ASDs in the United States between 2000 and 2008. The figures show a steady rise in the prevalence of ASDs. In 2000, approximately 1 in 150 children were diagnosed with ASDs, and by 2008, 1 in 88 children were diagnosed with an ASD. The question of whether ASDs are actually increasing is a topic of considerable controversy, however. There has been speculation that the increased number of ASD cases is not due to the disorder actually become more prevalent but is instead a result of ASD diagnosis criteria become broader and practitioners become more attentive to seeking out and identifying early indicators of autism.

Data

Table 8.2 Prevalence of ASDs in Eight-year-old Children (2008)

		About 1 in every X Children
Overall		1 in 88
Gender	Boys	1 in 54
	Girls	1 in 252
Race	Non-Hispanic white	1 in 83
	Non-Hispanic black	1 in 98
	Asian-Pacific Islander	1 in 103
	Hispanic	1 in 126

Source: http://www.nimh.nih.gov/statistics/1AUT_CHILD.shtml

Analysis

Table 8.2 shows the prevalence of ASD in eight-year-old children, organized by gender and race. The data does not show the existence of significant differences in the prevalence of autism rates by race or ethnicity. However, there are significant gender differences, with boys being five times more likely than girls to be affected by autism. Researcher has not yet established a clear and certain reason for these gender differences. However, recent research suggests a possible genetic component since it has been show that males who carry specific genetic alterations on their X chromosome have an elevated risk for developing ASD.

DISCUSSION QUESTIONS

1. It has been suggested that certain vaccines might be a causal factor in the development of autism. Do you find arguments suggesting a causal relationship between vaccines and autism to be persuasive? Why or why not?
2. Autism is more five times more common in boys than girls. What are some possible reasons for the gender differences?

3. Research shows an upward trend in the number of diagnosed cases of autism. Do you believe that the disorder is becoming more prevalent or that there have been such improvements in diagnosing autism that it only seems like the actual number of cases is increasing?
4. While there is no cure for autism, early intervention strategies can be effective in helping a child with an ASD to be less symptomatic? What do you think are some of the most useful interventions for a young child affected with ASD?
5. Many children who are diagnosed with ASDs have the opportunity to have early intervention services in specialized schools. Do you think it is most effective for children with ASDs to received early intervention services in specialized institutions or should efforts be directed toward enabling these students to attend mainstream educational institutions?

9

AUTOIMMUNE DISEASES

INTRODUCTION

Understanding Autoimmune Diseases

The term autoimmune diseases is used to describe a disorder that occurs when healthy body tissue is mistakenly destroyed by the immune system. There are over 80 different types of autoimmune disorders affecting 5–8% of Americans.

The immune system's white blood cells, regulatory T-cells, and antibodies normally fight harmful antigens, such as bacteria, viruses, toxins, and cancer cells. When an individual contracts an autoimmune disease, their immune system cannot distinguish between healthy body tissue and antigens. The cause of this inability to recognize healthy tissue is currently unknown. Similar to a hypersensitivity reaction that occurs in allergic conditions, this leads the immune system to attack and destroy normal body tissues. Some theories state that certain antigens or drugs trigger the change, while others focus on chemical and environmental causes.

The acquiring of an autoimmune disease may lead to the abnormal growth of an organ or changes in organ function, in addition to the deterioration of body tissues. Multiple organs and tissues can be affected by the disease, including blood vessels, connective tissues, endocrine glands, joints, muscles, red blood cells, and skin. Autoimmune diseases are classified as localized or organ-specific, in which a direct organ is affected, or they are classified as systemic or non-organ-specific, in which the entire body is affected. Common organ-specific diseases include Type I diabetes, Hashimoto's thyroiditis, Graves' disease, and Addison's disease. Common non-organ-specific diseases include rheumatoid arthritis, multiple sclerosis, lupus, and myasthenia gravis. It is also possible for an individual to suffer from multiple autoimmune diseases at one time and research suggests that once an individual suffers from an autoimmune disease, they are more likely to become afflicted by one or more additional autoimmune diseases.

Symptoms

The symptoms of autoimmune diseases vary based on the disease and the location of the abnormal immune response. However, there are certain symptoms that are common among autoimmune diseases. These include fatigue, fever, and a general ill feeling. The symptoms often fluctuate between periods of remission and flare-ups. Additional common symptoms include:

- Joint/muscle pain
- Skin rashes
- Numbness/tingling in hands and feet
- Changes in weight
- Hair loss
- Shortness of breath
- Recurrent miscarriage
- Depression
- Swollen glands
- Food allergies

Diagnosis

Autoimmune diseases can be difficult to diagnose and many individuals suffer for years before a proper diagnosis is made. Diagnosis should be determined by a health care professional who can distinguish the different symptoms related to each specific disease. Many diseases pose similar symptoms, so it may be difficult to distinguish which autoimmune disease one presents.

Tests to diagnose the autoimmune disease may be administered. Common tests used for diagnosis will examine antinuclear antibody tests, which look for the antibodies that are attacking cells in the body; autoantibody tests, which examine antibodies specific to an individual's tissues; complete blood counts, which measure the amount of red blood cells, white blood cells, hemoglobin, and hematocrit; C-reactive protein, which is produced by the liver and causes inflammation; and erythrocyte sedimentation rate, which measures how much inflammation is in the body. Family medical history should also be examined.

Risk Factors

The cause of autoimmune diseases is currently unknown, so there are no preventative measures available. It is thought that people with certain genes are more likely to acquire autoimmune diseases, as they often run in families. Both sexes and various age groups can be affected by autoimmune diseases; however, 75% of individuals affected are females, most during their childbearing years. African Americans, Hispanics, and Native Americans also tend to have an increased risk.

Treatment

Most autoimmune diseases are chronic; however, with the right treatment, symptoms can be controlled. Similar to diagnosis, the methods of treatment depend on the autoimmune disease and its location in the body. There are currently no cures for autoimmune diseases, so the main goals of treatment are to reduce symptoms, control the autoimmune process, and maintain the body's ability to fight disease.

Some patients may require supplements to replace hormones or vitamins, while others may need blood transfusions or assistance with movement and daily functions. Immunosuppressive medications, corticosteroid drugs, and nonsteroidal anti-inflammatory drugs can be administered to control or reduce symptoms. Other methods that may alleviate symptoms focus on strengthening an individual's immune system, including diet changes, restraint from alcohol or drug use, exercise, limiting sun exposure, or alternative therapies.

DATA AND ANALYSES

Data

Table 9.1 Ratios of Autoimmune Disease Prevalence Among Genders: 2013

Autoimmune disease	Female: Male
Hashimoto's thyroiditis	10:1
Systemic lupus erythematosus	9:1
Sjogren's syndrome	9:1
Antiphospholipid syndrome—secondary	9:1
Primary biliary cirrhosis	9:1
Autoimmune hepatitis	8:1
Graves' disease	7:1
Scleroderma	3:1
Rheumatoid arthritis	2.5:1
Antiphospholipid syndrome—primary	2:1
Autoimmune thrombocytopenic purpura	2:1
Multiple sclerosis	2:1
Myasthenia gravis	2:1

Source: American Autoimmune Related Diseases Association. 2005."Autoimmune disease in women." Retrieved from: http://www.aarda.org/autoimmune-information/autoimmune-disease-in-women/

Analysis

In total, autoimmune diseases affect females three times more than males. Table 9.1 shows the certain diseases that tend to appear more often in females than males. Females have enhanced immune systems, which increases their resistance to infection; however, it also makes them more susceptible to acquiring autoimmune diseases. Additionally, most females are affected during their childbearing years, which leads to an increased risk of passing on the genes that make an individual more susceptible.

Data

Table 9.2 Prevalence of Selected Autoimmune Diseases: 2005

Autoimmune disease	Number of cases per 100,000 people
Rheumatoid arthritis	860
Psoriasis	380
Crohn's disease	201

Autoimmune disease	Number of cases per 100,000 people
Type I diabetes	192
Multiple sclerosis	58
Lupus	24

Source: Health Union. 2005. "RA Statistics." Retrieved from: http://rheumatoidarthritis. net/what-is-ra/ra-statistics/

Analysis

Table 9.2 represents the prevalence of some of the most common autoimmune diseases in the United States. Rheumatoid arthritis proves to be one of the leading diseases, followed by other conditions such as psoriasis, Crohn's disease, and Type I (insulin-dependent) diabetes.

DISCUSSION QUESTIONS

1. What causes females to have enhanced immune systems? What measures can be taken to prevent the immune systems from attacking and destroying body tissues and organs?
2. What genes are responsible for autoimmune diseases? How can females prevent passing on these harmful genes to their children?
3. Why do some autoimmune diseases have a greater prevalence in females than others?
4. Should a cure for the most prevalent autoimmune diseases be focused on, rather than a general cure for all autoimmune diseases? Additionally, which autoimmune diseases tend to pose the most chronic prognosis?
5. What is the reason for the decrease in rheumatoid arthritis cases each year? What treatments are most commonly used for this disease, and are they administered for all autoimmune diseases? If so, how do the results compare?

10

BREAST CANCER

INTRODUCTION

Understanding Breast Cancer

Cancer originates in cells when there is an abnormality in the regeneration process. Cancer cells can be new cells that form when the body no longer requires them, or old damaged cells that do not die regularly. Both conditions lead to a mass of cells known as a tumor or lump. Tumors can be benign, noncancerous, or malignant, cancerous.

Inside each breast are 15–20 lobes, made up of lobules that contain milk-producing glands. Ducts are thin tubes that carry milk from the lobules to the nipple. The most common type of breast cancer is ductal carcinoma, which originates in the ducts and affects about seven out of ten women with breast cancer. Lobular carcinoma is another type of breast cancer that originate in the lobules, affecting about one out of ten women with breast cancer. Some women may have a mixture of both types.

Breast cancer can be invasive, spreading from the breast ducts or lobules to surrounding tissues. Most commonly, breast cancer cells enter the lymphatic vessels and begin to grow in lymph nodes.

Symptoms

The most common symptom of breast cancer is a lump or mass in the breast, also known as a tumor. Other symptoms include:

- Swelling of the breast
- Skin irritation
- Breast or nipple pain
- Nipple retraction
- Redness of the breast
- Thickening of the nipple or breast skin
- Nipple discharge, other than milk

Symptoms worsen as the cancer spreads and advances through the stages of breast cancer. The stages of breast cancer are based off of the size of the tumor and whether it has spread to other parts of the body. They are classified by roman numeral and letters. For example, stage IA occurs when the tumor is less than two centimeters wide, but the cells have not spread to the lymph nodes.

Diagnosis

Screening exams can be used for early detection of breast cancer in individuals who do not present any symptoms of breast cancer. Professionals often use mammograms, clinical breast exams, or magnetic resonance imaging (MRI) for early detection tests. Self-breast exams are also important in detecting breast cancer during the early stages and preventing growth or spreading of cancer cells.

If an individual does pose breast cancer symptoms, a professional will consider their current symptoms, prevalence of risk factors, prior health conditions, and family history. If breast cancer is suspected, tests will be administered to determine whether the tumor is malignant, the size of the tumor, and the spread of the cancer cells. Tests used to diagnose breast cancer include:

- Diagnostic mammogram: X-ray of the breast
- MRI: Magnet, radio waves are used to make a series of detailed images of areas inside the body
- Breast ultrasound: High-energy sound waves bounce off internal tissues or organs to make echoes, which form a picture of body tissues

- Blood chemistry studies: Blood samples are checked to measure certain substances released into the bloody by organs and tissues
- Biopsy: Removing cells or tissues to view under a microscope
    - Excisional biopsy: Removing an entire lump of tissue
    - Incisional biopsy: Removing part of a lump or a sample of tissue
    - Core biopsy: Removing tissue using a wide needle
    - Fine-needle aspiration biopsy: Removing tissue or fluid with a thin needle

After these studies, if an individual is diagnosed with breast cancer, further studies may be done to study the growth and recurrence of the cancer cells, as well as to determine the best method of treatment. These tests include:

- Estrogen and progesterone receptor status
- Human epidermal growth factor type 2 receptor status (HER2)

Risk Factors

It is not yet known what causes cells to become cancerous, yet researchers have found the most connections to hormones and genetics.

Some women may have no apparent risk factors and develop breast cancer, while others with multiple risk factors may never develop breast cancer. Common risk factors for breast cancer include:

- Gender: The main risk factor of breast cancer, as females are affected almost 100 times more than males due to estrogen and progesterone's promotion of breast cancer cell growth
- Aging: Breast cancer increases with age, as two out of three females with the disease are aged 55 or older
- Genetics: Mutations in specific genes lead to an increased risk of breast cancer
- Family history: Individuals with a family history of breast cancer have an almost doubled risk of developing the disease
- Personal history: Individuals who have previously been diagnosed with breast cancer have a higher risk of recurrence or development in the other breast

- Race: White women are slightly more likely to develop breast cancer than African Americans; however, African American women are more likely to die from the disease and present it at a younger age
- Pre-existing benign conditions
- Lifestyle factors: Having children, taking birth control, drinking alcohol, being overweight, and several other lifestyle factors may increase the risk of breast cancer
- Many other unclear or controversial factors are still being researched and discussed

Treatment

There are various treatment options for breast cancer, including surgery, radiation therapy, hormone therapy, chemotherapy, or targeted therapy. Most individuals will have some form of surgery combined with other treatments. Treatment is usually determined by the size and stage of the breast cancer, whether the tumor has hormone receptors, whether the tumor has an increased level of HER2, and the individual's general health.

Surgery options include:

- Lumpectomy: Removal of cancerous tissue, as well as surrounding normal tissue
- Mastectomy: Removal of the entire breast
- Modified radical mastectomy: Removal of the entire breast and lymph nodes under the arm

Radiation therapy options include:

- External beam radiation: Over a period of five to six weeks, radiation is focused from a machine on the cancerous part of the body
- Internal radiation therapy: Also known as brachytherapy, radioactive substances are sealed in needles, seeds, wires, or catheters and placed directly into or near the cancer

Systemic therapy options include:

- Targeted therapy: Tratuzumab, an antibody, is administered to target and slow the production of the HER2 protein
- Chemotherapy: A combination of drugs used depending on the stage of cancer

- Hormone therapy: Tamoxifen and Toremifene, as well as other aromatase inhibitors, are administered to lower estrogen levels or block the effects of estrogen

DATA AND ANALYSES

Data

Table 10.1 Five-year Relative Survival Rate Determined by Various Stages of Breast Cancer

Stage of breast cancer	Size of the tumor	Possible spread of the tumor	5-year relative survival rate
0	<2 cm	None	100%
I	<2 cm	Lymph nodes	100%
II	0–5 cm	Underarm lymph nodes or lymph nodes behind the breast bone	93%
III	Any size	Underarm lymph nodes, lymph nodes behind the breast bone, or lymph nodes surrounding the collarbone	72%
IV	Any size	Any other part of the body, such as brain, lungs, bones, etc.	22%

Source: American Cancer Society. 2014. "Breast cancer." Retrieved from: http://www.cancer.org/cancer/breastcancer/detailedguide/breast-cancer-detailed-guide-toc

Analysis

Survival rates are used to discuss an individual's prognosis, or outlook on recovery. The five-year survival rates refer to the percentage of patients who live at least five years after being diagnosed with cancer. Many patients go on to live much longer than five years after diagnosis. To obtain five-year survival rates, doctors examine individuals who were treated at least five years ago. Survival rates are based on large samples of individuals who had the disease; however, they cannot predict individual outcomes. As improvements in treatment become more available, prognoses may improve.

Substage results are not obtained, such as IA and IB, yet they can be assumed to be relatively similar to the rate for the categorized stage, such as I or II. Substages categorized with an A, such as IA, can be assumed to have a slightly better prognosis than stage I, while substages categorized with a B, such as IB, can be assumed to have a slightly worse prognosis than stage I.

The data in Table 10.1 demonstrates that as stages advance, the prognosis for a positive outcome worsens. This is due to the fact that as a patient advances through higher stages of breast cancer, the cancer becomes apparent in more parts of their body. Individuals with stages 0–II cancer tend to have a relatively positive prognosis, as the tumor remains relatively small and may have only spread to the underarm lymph nodes. In stage III, the prognosis worsens as the tumor can be any size and may have spread to the underarm lymph nodes, the lymph nodes behind the breastbone, or the lymph nodes surrounding the collarbone. Lastly, stage IV poses the worst possible prognosis, as the tumor can be any size and has spread to other parts of the body at this point, such as the bones, brain, or lungs.

Data

Table 10.2 U.S. Cancer Deaths vs. Cancer Research in 2010

Type of cancer	Annual death rate per 100,000	Annual amount spent on research per million dollars
Lung	51.7	246.9
Prostate	23.6	293.9
Breast	23.4	599.5
Colon	17.1	264.2
Pancreas	10.8	89.7
Ovary	8.5	110.1
Leukemia	7.2	220.6
Non-Hodgkin's lymphoma	6.7	130.9
Liver	5.3	70.3
Esophagus	4.4	28.8

Source: Goodman, J. 2010. "Cancer deaths vs. cancer research." National Center for Policy Analysis. Retrieved from: http://healthblog.ncpa.org/cancer-deaths-vs-cancer-research/

Analysis

The National Cancer Institute examined the ten types of cancer that produce the most deaths in the United States, compared to the amount of money that is spent on research for that particular cancer. Death rates vary by gender and ethnicity; however, this study looked at overall rates.

Table 10.2 shows that lung cancer is responsible for the most deaths by cancer in the United States, doubling the second-leading types of cancer, which are prostate cancer and breast cancer. Contrastingly, the National Cancer Institute and the American Cancer Society both devote the most amount of money to funding breast cancer research. The amount of funds devoted to breast cancer research more than doubles the amount of funds devoted to lung cancer research and prostate cancer research.

DISCUSSION QUESTIONS

1. What preventative measures can be taken to prevent breast cancer from advancing to stage IV, as this type of cancer poses the worst prognosis?
2. What risk factors have an effect on the stage and prognosis of breast cancer? Do these risk factors speed up or inhibit the progression of the tumor's growth?
3. If the amount of research funds for breast cancer is almost double that of lung cancer and prostate cancer, which both contribute to more deaths in the United States, why is breast cancer still the third-most deadly form of cancer?
4. What are the funds for breast cancer research focusing on—prevention, treatment, etc.? Is there a better way to distribute these funds?
5. Why are some cancers more common than others?

11

BREASTFEEDING

INTRODUCTION

Understanding Breastfeeding

After babies transition from the womb to the world, they need to be properly nourished to survive and thrive. In such a crucial stage of development, milk is usually the first and perhaps the most important part of a child's early diet. For most babies and their mothers, breastfeeding is the most popular, convenient, and natural option for providing the nutrition a baby needs as it continues to grow. Breastfeeding involves nursing an infant with milk from a female human breast instead of using manufactured food such as baby formula.

Process

Lactation is the process that makes breastfeeding possible. During the second or third trimesters of a mother's pregnancy, certain hormones are automatically produced to induce milk production in the grapelike alveoli and ducts embedded within the breasts. Some of these hormones, like progesterone and estrogen, remain at high levels during pregnancy to prevent lactation from occurring before birth, but drop sharply at delivery to trigger flow. The first breast milk that a mother produces is called colostrum. It is thick and yellow, providing hormones and antibodies to help infants fill up quickly and protect them from infection.

To breastfeed directly, a mother can simply position her baby's mouth on her nipple and allow them to use their natural reflex to suck the breast milk from the milk ducts while she supports her breast. Mothers can begin breastfeeding in the delivery room when their baby is born, and most mothers in the United States usually begin to wean their children off breastfeeding when they reach 6 months of age. However, some mothers continue to breastfeed until their infant is one-year-old and beyond, supplementing the breast milk with solid foods to provide them with an even more complete package of nutrition. Regardless of a child's age, feedings usually take less than an hour and are normally conducted 8–12 times a day.

To breastfeed indirectly, some mothers opt to use a breast pump to extract milk from the breast into containers and feed to their child at a later time. This option is ideal if a mother is traveling, at work, or in a location where she cannot breastfeed her child directly.

Benefits

As a natural process, there are several short- and long-term advantages to breastfeeding that other methods of nourishing infants do not offer. When babies are breastfed, they can benefit from:

- More resilient immune systems
- Fewer respiratory infections
- Fewer urinary tract infections
- Improved gastrointestinal development
- Lower probability of obesity
- Lower probability of cardiovascular disease
- Lower probability of diabetes

Infants being breastfed are not the only ones who can benefit from the practice. There are also many advantages for mothers who decide to breastfeed. These include:

- Intimate bonding time with the infant
- More economical way to provide nutrition
- Lower risk of breast cancer
- Lower risk of ovarian cancer

- Lower risk of diabetes
- Lower risk of postpartum depression

Drawbacks

Unfortunately, advantages of breastfeeding also come with disadvantages that may pose challenges to new and experienced mothers alike. Mothers who breastfeed might experience:

- Sore nipples
- Engorgement of breasts
- Breast infection, called mastitis
- Physical discomfort
- Vaginal dryness

Aside from these physical drawbacks, a mother must also pay special attention to her diet and anything she ingests—generally, the same way she had to during her pregnancy. Foods, drinks, substances, and medications that a mother ingests can all be passed to a child through her breast milk and cause discomfort, indigestion, or illness in the child.

DATA AND ANALYSES

Data

Table 11.1 Prevalence in Number and Percentage of U.S. Mothers Who Ever Breastfed Based on Race and Ethnicity, 1992, 1995, 1998, 2001

	Ever breastfed	
	Number	%
Non-Hispanic white mothers		
1992	23,206	33.3%
1995	21,602	35.9%
1998	19,352	44.0%
2001	19,955	49.5%
Non-Hispanic black mothers		
1992	32,008	13.8%
1995	28,474	17.2%
1998	25,234	23.2%
2001	18,770	30.8%

(Continued)

Table 11.1 Prevalence in Number and Percentage of U.S. Mothers Who Ever Breastfed Based on Race and Ethnicity, 1992, 1995, 1998, 2001 (*Continued*)

	Ever breastfed	
	Number	%
Hispanic mothers		
1992	17,784	36.1%
1995	20,931	43.9%
1998	20,260	50.4%
2001	20,811	62.7%

Source: Centers for Disease Control and Prevention, Who and when: Is breastfeeding prevalence increasing or decreasing among racial and ethnic groups over time? Retrieved from: http://www.cdc.gov/pednss/how_to/interpret_data/case_studies/breastfeeding/who_and_when.htm

Analysis

Table 11.1 illustrates the relationship between breastfeeding in non-Hispanic white mothers, non-Hispanic black mothers, and Hispanic mothers in 1992, 1995, 1998, and 2001.

The number of non-Hispanic white mothers who ever breastfed decreased from 23,206 in 1992 to 19,955 in 2001, while the percentage increased from 33.3% to 49.5%. A similar trend was observed with non-Hispanic black mothers who ever breastfed, with a number decreasing from 32,008 in 1992 to 18,770 in 2001, and a percentage increasing from 13.8% in 1992 to 30.8% in 2001.

Hispanic mothers who ever breastfed showed an increase in both categories, with numbers starting with 17,784 in 1992 and ending 20,811 in 2001, and percentages rising from 36.1% in 1992 to 62.7% in 2001.

Data

Table 11.2 Rates of Any and Exclusive Breastfeeding of Children in the United States With Age of Breastfed Child, 2010

	Breastfeeding (n = 84,396)	Exclusive breastfeeding (n = 8,287)
At birth	76.5 ± 1.6	Data not available
7 days	75.6 ± 1.6	54.1 ± 1.9
14 days	74.8 ± 1.6	52.3 ± 1.9

	Breastfeeding (n = 84,396)	Exclusive breastfeeding (n = 8,287)
21 days	73.1 ± 1.6	50.0 ± 1.9
28 days	72.4 ± 1.7	49.2 ± 1.9
42 days	68.6 ± 1.7	43.8 ± 1.9
1 month	72.0 ± 1.7	48.6 ± 1.9
2 months	66.7 ± 1.8	42.5 ± 1.9
3 months	62.5 ± 1.8	37.7 ± 1.9
4 months	56.6 ± 1.9	29.1 ± 1.8
5 months	51.8 ± 1.9	21.4 ± 1.6
6 months	49.0 ± 1.9	16.4 ± 1.5
7 months	40.6 ± 1.9	Data not available
8 months	37.3 ± 1.9	Data not available
9 months	34.8 ± 1.9	Data not available
10 months	32.0 ± 1.8	Data not available
11 months	29.0 ± 1.8	Data not available
12 months	27.0 ± 1.8	Data not available
18 months	9.4 ± 1.2	Data not available

Note: Numbers are expressed through the formula: (percentage +/– half 95% confidence interval).

Source: Centers for Disease Control and Prevention, Breastfeeding among U.S. Children born 2001–2011, CDC National Immunization Survey. Retrieved from: http://www.cdc.gov/breastfeeding/data/nis_data/index.htm

Analysis

Table 11.2 shows the prevalence of two kinds of breastfeeding at different ages, starting from a child's birth to 18 months old, taken from a 2010 study. In general, the numbers show that breastfeeding exclusively with breast milk has been consistently less popular than breastfeeding with added liquids or solids at every age surveyed. In some cases, such as the five- and six-month checkpoints, the amount of children being breastfed in any way was double and triple the amount of those being exclusively breastfed, respectively.

The amount of children being exclusively breastfed decreased significantly from 54.1 ± 1.9 when the child was seven days old to 16.4 ± 1.5 when the child was six months old. After six months, mothers tend to wean their children off of exclusive breast milk so they will stop lactating, which might explain why a significant rate of data is not available beyond this age group. Although the range of data for breastfeeding with added liquids and solids also shows a decrease, there was a more incremental decline.

DISCUSSION QUESTIONS

1. Most mothers begin to wean their children from their breast milk by the six-month or one-year age checkpoint. Is it possible for mothers to breastfeed years after their child is born? Why might this not be the most effective supply of nutrition for an older child?

2. Some women are criticized for breastfeeding their children in public places, including at restaurants or at the office. What laws or programs do you know of that are in place to either protect or guard against women breastfeeding children in front of others?

3. Breastfeeding mothers are encouraged to watch what they eat and to make healthy choices when it comes to filling their plates. What foods, drinks, or substances would be considered unhealthy choices for a breastfeeding mother, and how might they affect the milk she produces for her baby?

4. Mothers tend to find it easier to lose pregnancy and pre-pregnancy weight when they are breastfeeding their babies. What is so different about this period of time that can influence the size of a mother's waistline?

5. Table 11.1 shows that the number of non-Hispanic white mothers and non-Hispanic black mothers who have ever breastfed has decreased over time, while the percentage of them has increased over time. Why might this be?

12

CALORIE CONSUMPTION

INTRODUCTION

Calories are the basic energy unit that allows living beings to function. Consuming nutrients through the ingestion of food provides individuals with the calories they need in order for their bodies to function while at rest and while performing activities, including strenuous physical exertion.

Calorie consumption also plays an important role in a person's body mass and weight. Consuming too many calories and not burning off enough of them through physical exertion, such as exercise, can make someone obese, whereas not eating enough or burning too many calories through excessive physical exertion can result in an individual being underweight and suffering from nutritional deficiencies. To remain healthy, individuals should attain an understanding of how many calories their bodies need and then monitor how many calories they consume and how many they burn off.

Balancing Your Calorie Count

Calories are stored in food primarily as three types of nutrients: carbohydrates, proteins, and fats. Proteins and carbohydrates tend to have four calories per gram while fats have nine, making them a higher source of calories. Individuals only need a certain number of calories per day, which means that if one consume more calories per day then their body needs and fails to burn off those calories through physical activity, that individual will typically gain weight.

A pound of fat is roughly 3,500 calories. Losing weight is not as simple as getting on a treadmill and running until the "calories burned" number reads 3,500. In fact, this is very unhealthy, as if you eat less than 40–50% of the calories you need in one day, your body will go into starvation mode, where all calories are converted to fat to protect the organs and your health begins to decline.

Someone looking to lose weight can cut out about 500–1,000 calories per day, depending on their original weight and goal weight. It is best to do this under the guidance of a health care professional, such as a nutritionists or dietician, who can make sure your sources of calories are healthy enough to support your body. To boost the effects of reduced caloric intake as one endeavors to lose weight, it can be helpful to increase general physical activity and to also introduce an exercise program. This will increase the number of calories that the body utilizes. When combining increased physical activity with reduced calorie intake, however, one must remain mindful of overall caloric needs and ensure that, while losing weight, one is consuming sufficient nutrients and calories to remain healthy.

When someone begins to lose weight, they often lose a combination of fat, lean tissue, and water, which is why results can be misleading at first. It is important to exercise to make sure that you gain muscle instead of lose it, as muscle helps keep off fat and burn more calories, even at rest. Also, once you have lost weight, you will need to consume fewer calories than you did before, meaning that those who go back to old eating habits may rapidly regain the weight they lost.

Ways to Reduce Calorie Intake

With the variety and number of processed foods that contain high amounts of fats and sugars increasingly on the rise, it is important to make sure you are getting your calories from healthy sources and consuming the proper amount of food.

One good way to do this is to eat small portions. By dividing daily caloric intake into small portions, you allow your body to feel full faster, and may reduce the likelihood of overeating. Measuring food to keep track of portion size can be very helpful, as can eating with friends and family. Studies show that those who eat in social groups eat less than those who do not, while eating in front of the television can lead to eating more servings, larger portions, and less healthy food.

Another strategy is to switch one unhealthy food choice with one healthier choice. Foods like fruits and vegetables are not only lower in calories, they are full of fiber, which leads to feeling fuller faster. Switching soda, juice, or alcohol for water is another easy way to do this, since those "empty" calories (calories from something that has no nutritional benefit) will be cut out of your diet. Similarly, taking less sugar and milk in a morning cup of coffee can help a great deal in reducing one's daily caloric consumption.

Finally, as noted above, it will also be important to increase one's activity level. Not only does exercise burn many more calories during the period that you are active (as opposed to if you were sitting on a couch), but it keeps burning more calories for up to 48 hours after. That time period is also one that will be spent not eating; some report a temptation to eat junk food while reading or watching TV, but it is difficult to indulge in such things while exercising.

Experts report many other tips and tricks to help control your daily calorie count, such as pacing while on the phone or tapping your foot while on the computer, doing sit-ups or using a stationary cardio machine while watching TV, leaving about 25% of your food on your plate for leftovers, and not having meals "family style," where the serving bowls are placed in the middle of the table, inviting people back for extra helpings.

DATA AND ANALYSES

Data

Table 12.1 Calories Burned per Hour Based on Physical Activity: United States, 2006

Moderate physical activity	Calories burned per hour
Hiking	370
Light gardening/yard work	330
Dancing	330
Golf (walking and carrying clubs)	330
Bicycling (less than 10 mph)	290
Walking (3.5 mph)	280
Weight lifting (light workout)	220
Stretching	180

(Continued)

Table 12.1 Calories Burned per Hour Based on Physical Activity: United States, 2006 (*Continued*)

Moderate physical activity	Calories burned per hour
Vigorous physical activity	
Running/jogging	590
Bicycling (more than 10 mph)	590
Swimming (slow freestyle laps)	510
Aerobics	480
Walking (4.5 mph)	460
Heavy yard work (chopping wood, for example)	440
Weight lifting (vigorous workout)	440
Basketball (vigorous)	440

Source: National Heart, Blood, and Lung Institute, 2006.

Analysis

Based on a 154-pound person, Table 12.1 presents the average number of calories that will be burned during an hour of various physical activities. A lighter person will burn fewer calories, while a heavier person will burn more calories per hour. Additionally, whether the weight is made up of fat or muscle determines how many calories are burned. A pound of fat only contributes to two calories burned while a pound of muscle contributes to 50 calories burned.

Low-impact sports, or those that do not raise your heart rate much, burn fewer calories per hour, such as walking at three miles per hour or swimming. Exercises that require a high heart rate, such as running at ten miles per hour, prompt a high rate of calories being burned. This is because such activities not only engage the body's life-support functions, like breathing and heart rate, and cause them to increase significantly, but they activate the metabolism and cause you to build muscle, which prolongs your use of calories.

Data

Table 12.2 Estimated Calorie Requirements for Gender and Age Group Based on Physical Activity Level: United States, 2013

Gender	Age group	Sedentary	Moderately active	Active
Female	4–8	1,200	1,400–1,600	1,400–1,800
	9–13	1,600	1,600–2,000	1,800–2,000
	14–18	1,800	2,000	2,400

Gender	Age group	Sedentary	Moderately active	Active
	19–30	2,000	2,000–2,200	2,400
	31–50	1,800	2,000	2,200
	51+	1,600	1,800	2,000–2,200
Male	4–8	1,400	1,400–1,600	1,600–2,000
	9–13	1,800	1,800–2,200	2,000–2,600
	14–18	2,200	2,400–2,800	2,800–3,200
	19–30	2,400	2,600–2,800	3,000
	31–50	2,200	2,400–2,600	2,800–3,000
	51+	2,000	2,200–2,400	2,400–2,800

Source: National Heart, Blood, and Lung Institute, 2013.

Analysis

Table 12.2 presents the average amount of calories that an individual should consume per day to maintain a healthy body weight, based on gender, age, and physical activity level. Sedentary activity levels include only light physical activity associated with daily life. Moderately active activity levels include physical activity that is equivalent to walking about 1.5–3 miles per day at 3–4 miles per hour in addition to the light physical activity of daily life. Active activity levels include physical activity equivalent to walking more than 3 miles per day at 3–4 miles per hour in addition to the light physical activity of daily life. Evidently, required caloric intake differs between genders, as males require more calories than females. Additionally, age factors into caloric intake, as younger and older individuals require fewer calories than young adults and middle-aged individuals. Furthermore, the largest factor of calorie consumption is physical activity levels, as people who exert more energy throughout the day will require a greater amount of calories. In order to lose weight, one should reduce the number of calories they need per day by about 500, leading to a 3,500-calorie loss over the coming week.

DISCUSSION QUESTIONS

1. As many as four out of five Americans report wanting to be healthier, but having no idea how many calories they should eat a day, or even what calories are. Do you believe enough is done to educate people on this topic?
2. Eating out, whether at a fast food place or a sit-down restaurant, can often result in the consumption of excess calories.

It can often be difficult to guess calorie count in such food, and a study showed that even most professional dieticians cannot do that accurately. What can be done to make sure consumers know what they are eating?

3. Many health issues come about from myths and misconceptions about dietary needs, but some believe the myths as opposed to facts. How can we make sure people not only receive proper nutritional education, but understand it?

4. Fad diets, like the grapefruit diet, and crash diets, where people eat fewer than 1,000 calories a day, are very popular, despite being dangerous and ineffective.

5. Some people consciously do not follow nutritional guidelines, eating unhealthy foods that have huge amounts of calories or taking in empty calories through sugary or alcoholic drinks. Should these people, who knowingly damage their bodies, be given the same consideration for medical treatment as someone who tries to take care of his or health?

13

CARDIOVASCULAR DISEASE

INTRODUCTION

Understanding Cardiovascular Disease

The heart is divided into two sides: one side produces oxygen-rich blood to circulate throughout the body, and the other holds oxygen-poor blood. The right side of the heart pumps blood to the lungs through the pulmonary arteries to supply it with oxygen. The oxygen-rich blood then enters the left side of the heart and is pumped throughout the body. Each side of the heart contains an atrium and a ventricle; altogether there are four one-way valves that keep the blood moving. A beating heart contracts, known as systole, and relaxes, known as diastole.

The causes of cardiovascular disease vary on the type of disease:

- Coronary artery disease: This disease of refers to damage caused by atherosclerosis, which is a buildup of fat in the arteries. The arteries carry oxygen-rich blood from the heart throughout the body. When there is a buildup of fatty plaque, blood flow is restricted.

- Heart arrhythmia: This disease refers to abnormal heart rhythms in which the heart's electrical impulses may not start or travel properly.
- Heart defects: This disease usually develops before a baby is born. Heart defects can begin to form about a month after conception when the heart begins to develop. However, defects can also occur as people age and their heart structures change.
- Cardiomyopathy: This disease consists of the thickening or enlarging of the heart muscle. The cause is unknown, yet there are three distinct types:
  - Dilated cardiomyopathy: The most common type of cardiomyopathy, in which the left ventricle becomes enlarged, weakening the pumping ability and reducing blood flow.
  - Hypertrophic cardiomyopathy: Abnormal growth or thickening of the heart muscle affects the left ventricle, shrinking the size of the pumping chamber and causing a weakened ability to pump blood throughout the body.
  - Restrictive cardiomyopathy: The heart muscle hardens so that the heart cannot properly expand and fill with blood in between heartbeats.
- Heart infection: This disease refers to when a toxin, such as a bacterium, virus or chemical reaches the heart muscle.
  - Common bacterium conditions are pericarditis, endocarditis, and myocarditis. Endocarditis can be caused by bacteria entering the bloodstream through everyday activities, while myocarditis may be caused by a live bacterium like ticks.
  - Common heart infections are caused by viruses such as influenza, gastrointestinal infections, mononucleosis, and sexually transmitted diseases.
  - Other infections may be caused by parasites, medication including antibiotics like penicillin, illegal substances like cocaine, and other diseases.
- Valvular heart disease: This disease affects the four one-way valves that direct blood flow.

Symptoms

Symptoms vary based on the type of cardiovascular disease.

- Coronary artery disease: Chest pain, shortness of breath, shoulder or arm pain, numbness, weakness or coldness in legs and arms

- Heart arrhythmia: Fluttering in the chest, racing or slow heartbeat, chest pain, shortness of breath, lightheadedness, dizziness, fainting
- Heart defects: As an infant, a patient may have pale gray or blue skin; swelling in the legs, abdomen or around the eyes; or shortness of breath during infancy feedings, leading to poor weight gain. Later in childhood, symptoms may present as being easily short of breath, tiring during exercise, built-up fluid in the heart or lungs, and swelling in the hands, ankles, and feet
- Cardiomyopathy: Breathlessness, swelling of legs, ankles or feet, bloating of the abdomen with fluid, fatigue, irregular or rapid heartbeat, dizziness, fainting
- Heart infection: Fever, short of breath, fatigue, swelling in the legs or abdomen, changes in heart rhythm, dry, persistent cough, and skin rash
- Valvular disease: Fatigue, short of breath, irregular heartbeat, swollen ankles or feet, chest pain, and fainting

Diagnosis

Different tests will be used for diagnosis depending on what condition doctors think is present. In addition to performing a physical exam and asking about family history, tests to diagnose heart disease include:

- Blood tests: Test for substances that indicate cardiovascular disease and checks cholesterol, triglycerides, and blood cell counts
- Chest X-ray: Shows an image of the heart, lungs, and blood vessels to reveal if the heart is enlarged, which is a sign of some forms of cardiovascular disease
- Electrocardiogram (ECG): Probes on the chest record electrical impulses that make the heart beat, helping detect irregularities in the heart's rhythm and structure
- Holter monitoring: Portable device that records heart rhythms continuously for 24–72 hours, detecting irregularities that cannot be found in a regular ECG exam
- Echocardiogram: Ultrasound of the chest that shows detailed images of the heart's structure and function
- Cardiac catheterization: X-ray images on a monitor help doctors guide a tube through the arteries to the heart where

pressures in the chambers can be measured and dye can be injected to see blood flow through the heart vessels and valves

- Heart biopsy: A tiny sample is removed during catheterization if heart inflammation is suspected
- Cardiac computerized tomography (CT) scan: Checks for heart failure and arrhythmias, as well as calcium buildups
- Cardiac magnetic resonance imaging (MRI): Radio waves produce signals and heart images created

Risk Factors

General risk factors for cardiovascular diseases include:

- Age: As people get older, there is an increased risk of damage and narrowing of the arteries, or weakening of heart muscle
- Gender: Males are at greater risk, yet female risk increases after menopause
- Family history
- Smoking: Nicotine constricts blood vessels and carbon monoxide damages inner lining
- Diet: Diets high in fat, salt, and cholesterol increase the risk of cardiovascular diseases
- High blood pressure: Increases the risk of thickening or hardening of the arteries, affecting blood flow
- High cholesterol levels: Increases the risk of formation of plaque and hardening of the arteries
- Diabetes: Increases the risk of heart disease, obesity, and high blood pressure
- Obesity and lack of activity: Worsens other risk factors
- Poor hygiene: Not regularly washing hands, poor dental health, and other unhygienic habits increases the risk for bacterial or viral infections

Treatment

Treatments vary based on conditions, yet the main goal is to open narrowed arteries that cause cardiovascular disease symptoms. Depending on the severity of blockages, treatment options could include:

- Coronary artery disease:
  - Lifestyle changes: Patients may be asked to eat a low-fat and low-sodium diet, get at least 30 minutes of moderate exercise a day, quit smoking, and limit alcohol
  - Medications: Certain medications will aim to lower blood pressure and cholesterol and thin the blood
  - Medical procedures: A coronary angioplasty consists of inserting a catheter and threading a small balloon through it to the blocked artery. The balloon is then inflated to reopen the artery and a metal stent is placed for support
- Heart arrhythmia:
  - Vagal maneuvers: Acts that affect the nervous, such as holding one's breath, putting water on the face or coughing, will help control heartbeats
  - Medical procedures: Electrical cardioversion is used to reset the heart to a regular rhythm, or ablation catheters can be threaded to the inner heart and electrodes can be positioned on certain areas to destroy heart tissue that is creating a block
  - Pacemakers and implantable cardioverter-defibrillators (ICDs): Electrical impulses are emitted to regulate the heartbeat regulate heartbeat
  - Medical procedures: Open heart surgery
- Heart defect:
  - Medication: Medication will be used to treat congenital heart defects
  - Medical procedures: Special procedures with catheters, open heart surgery or heart transplants
- Cardiomyopathy:
  - Medication: Medication can improve the pumping ability of the heart
  - Pacemakers and ICDs
  - Medical procedures: Heart transplant
- Heart infection:
  - Medication: Antibiotics and medication to regulate heartbeats may be given
- Valvular heart disease:
  - Medication: Medication can help open blood vessels, lower cholesterol, reduce water retention, and thin the blood
  - Medical procedures: Balloon valvuloplasty is similar to a catheterization, but focuses on opening narrowed pulmonary valves to increase blood flow. Valve repair or valve replacement surgery may also be used

DATA AND ANALYSES

Data

Table 13.1 Leading Causes of Death: United States, 2010

Cause of death	Total deaths
Cardiovascular disease	596,577
Cancer	576,691
Chronic lower respiratory diseases	142,943
Stroke (cerebrovascular diseases)	128,932
Accidents (unintentional injuries)	126,438
Alzheimer disease	84,974
Diabetes	73,831
Influenza and pneumonia	53,826
Nephritis, nephrotic syndrome, and nephrosis	45,591
Intentional self-harm (suicide)	39,518

Source: Data from American Heart Association. 2013. "Men & cardiovascular disease." American Heart Association. Retrieved from: http://www.heart.org/idc/groups/heart-public/@wcm/@sop/@smd/documents/downloadable/ucm_319573.pdf

Analysis

Table 13.1 clarifies the severity of cardiovascular diseases as the leading cause of death in the United States, as cancer is the only other cause of death that results in similar rates. Cancer attributed to 576,691 deaths in 2010, while the third leading cause, chronic lower respiratory diseases, only caused 142, 943 deaths. The other causes of death that round out the top-five leading causes are stroke and accidents. All other causes of death that made the list of top-ten leading causes attributed to less than 100,000 deaths in 2010. Therefore, the data presents the importance of further research examining the top-two leading causes of death, heart disease, and cancer, and how the death rates can be lowered.

Data

Table 13.2 Percentage of Individuals With Reported Heart Disease by Stress Level: Adults, Ages 50–64, 2010

During the past 4 weeks, felt calm and peaceful	
Stress level during the past four weeks	Percentage of individuals with reported heart disease
All of the time	24.7%
Most of the time	21.6%

During the past 4 weeks, felt calm and peaceful	
Stress level during the past four weeks	Percentage of individuals with reported heart disease
Some of the time	14.1%
Little or none of the time	10.6%

Source: Carroll, W. & Miller, G.E. 2013. "Heart disease among near elderly Americans: Estimates for the U.S. civilian noninstitutionalized population, 2010." U.S. Department of Health & Human Services. Retrieved from: http://meps.ahrq.gov/data_files/ publications/st408/stat408.shtml

Analysis

In 2010, 16.8% of U.S. individuals aged 50–64 reported diagnoses of heart disease. In total, there is an estimated 60.5 million people that make up this population. Of the deaths in this population, over 90,000 were related to cardiovascular diseases, amounting to about 22% of total deaths. The U.S. Department of Health and Human Services conducted studies to examine specific risk factors and their relation to cardiovascular diseases. Specifically, the levels of stress that an individual experienced were compared with the prevalence of cardiovascular diseases. As shown in Table 13.2, the levels of stress that individuals experience directly relates to the percentage of cardiovascular disease diagnoses. Individuals who stated that they felt calm "all of the time" were the least likely to present a cardiovascular disease diagnosis.

In addition, further research found that individuals in poor or near-poor areas and low-income families were more likely to be diagnosed with cardiovascular diseases. Similarly, individuals with less than a high school education and individuals with only a high school degree were both more likely to be diagnosed. These risk factors may be directly related to an increase in stress, which lead to an increase in cardiovascular diseases.

DISCUSSION QUESTIONS

1. What caused the change in research findings regarding the prevalence of cardiovascular diseases among males and females? Why are females now accounting for more deaths from cardiovascular diseases than males?
2. How do the differences in risk factors affect the prevalence of cardiovascular diseases in males and females? Do certain risk factors have a higher relation to developing cardiovascular diseases?

3. What preventative measures can be taken to lessen the amounts of cardiovascular disease-related deaths? Why are cardiovascular diseases the leading cause of death in the United States?
4. Do other risk factors effect one's level of stress, which is directly related to cardiovascular diseases? Are some risk factors more closely related to cardiovascular diseases than others?
5. How do levels of stress and prevalence of cardiovascular diseases in individuals age 50–64 compare to other ages?

14

CERVICAL CANCER

INTRODUCTION

Understanding Cervical Cancer

As the part of the body that joins the uterus to the vagina with a muscular passageway, the cervix is a crucial part of the female reproductive system. For this reason, any damage or disease that the cervix experiences deals a major blow to its functionality during childbearing and menstruation. Cervical cancer, a gynecological cancer that attacks the cervix, is just one example of this kind of damage and disease.

When a woman participates in sexual intercourse, she risks contracting the sexually transmitted human papillomavirus. This virus is the most common infection of its kind in the reproductive tract and usually results in genital warts that cure themselves after a period of time. Although the virus does not necessarily lead to cervical cancer, constant infections can cause cells in the cervix to change into cervical cancer cells. When this occurs, the human papillomavirus strain is classified as "high risk," and the cervix is forced to fight against it. It is also worth mentioning that the most aggressive cervical cancer cells have the ability to spread to nearby areas of a woman's body.

Symptoms

Cervical cancer in its early stage of development does not show many symptoms. Instead, symptoms appear once the disease has progressed into its advanced stages and begun to attack nearby tissue. Some symptoms of cervical cancer include:

- Abnormal vaginal bleeding that occurs after vaginal intercourse, between periods, or after menopause
- Abnormal, heavy vaginal discharge that contains blood and emits a strong odor
- Pelvic pain
- Pain during vaginal intercourse

Diagnosis

Because the symptoms of cervical cancer are also common symptoms for other gynecological cancers—such as ovarian cancer, uterine cancer, vaginal cancer, and vulvar cancer—the only surefire way to diagnose cervical cancer is to consult a medical professional. Two screening tests, the Pap smear test and human papillomavirus test, are the main diagnostic tools used by doctors to identify cervical cancer and are extremely helpful in detecting cervical cancer before it progresses.

The first, the Pap smear test, is recommended for women between 21 and 65 years of age and is typically administered every three years. During the test, a doctor widens a woman's vagina with a special instrument called a speculum and takes a sample of cells from the cervix to analyze it for any cell changes or cancerous tissue.

For even more accurate results, women older than 30 years opt to co-test their Pap smear samples with the HPV test to check for the virus that causes cervical cancer.

Risk Factors

There are several risk factors associated with cervical cancer patients that increase the likelihood of contracting the disease. It is worth noting that although there are other risk factors, having a human papillomavirus infection in the cervix is the most common risk factor for cervical cancer and is the cause of an overwhelming majority of cervical cancer cases. The known risk factors for cervical cancer include:

- Having a human papillomavirus infection in the cervix
- Having sexually transmitted infections like chlamydia, gonorrhea, syphilis, or HIV/AIDs

- Giving birth to several children
- Having many sexual partners
- Beginning sexual activity at an early age
- Using contraceptives
- Smoking cigarettes
- Having a weak immune system

Treatment

Cervical cancer is a cancer that is easily treatable, especially when detected in its early stages. Whether the cancer is still mild or has become aggressive, treatment is usually directed to a gynecologic oncologist who specializes in monitoring and treating reproductive cancers in women.

There are three main kinds of treatment for patients suffering from cervical cancer, which include surgery, chemotherapy, and radiation. While surgery removes the cancerous tissue through an operation on the cervix and surrounding areas that the cancer has spread to, chemotherapy involves the use of oral or intravenous drugs to kill the disease. Radiation, on the other hand, aims special rays of high energy onto the cervix area in an effort to destroy the cancer. In general, the type of treatment recommended by the oncologist largely depends on the size and stage of the cancer.

In addition to the three standard kinds of treatment for cervical cancer, there are also complementary medicines that are used in addition to the treatment of choice and alternative medicines that are used as a substitute. These can include different forms of exercise and diet changes, like yoga sessions or vitamin supplements.

DATA AND ANALYSES

Data

Table 14.1 Incidence Rate of Top Ten Cancer Sites in Women of All Races and Ethnicities, White Women, and Asian/Pacific Islander Women in the United States, 2006–2010

Cancer site	Rate
All races	
1. Female breast	121.9
2. Lung and bronchus	55.3

(Continued)

**Table 14.1 Incidence Rate of Top Ten Cancer Sites in Women of All
Races and Ethnicities, White Women, and Asian/Pacific Islander
Women in the United States, 2006–2010** (*Continued*)

Cancer site	Rate
3. Colon and rectum	39.1
4. Corpus and uterus	24.6
5. Thyroid	18.5
6. Non-Hodgkin lymphoma	16.2
7. Melanomas of the skin	15.6
8. Ovary	12.3
9. Kidney and renal pelvis	11.2
10. Pancreas	10.7
White	
1. Female breast	123.2
2. Lung and bronchus	57.0
3. Colon and rectum	38.1
4. Corpus and uterus	25.1
5. Thyroid	19.5
6. Melanomas of the skin	17.9
7. Non-Hodgkin lymphoma	16.7
8. Ovary	12.7
9. Kidney and renal pelvis	11.3
10. Pancreas	10.4
Asian/Pacific Islander	
1. Female breast	84.2
2. Colon and rectum	30.9
3. Lung and bronchus	27.9
4. Thyroid	18.5
5. Corpus and uterus	16.8
6. Non-Hodgkin lymphoma	10.3
7. Stomach	9.0
8. Ovary	8.9
9. Pancreas	8.3
10. Liver and intrahepatic bile duct	8.0

Note: Rates are per 100,000 women and are age-adjusted to the 2000 United States standard
population.

Source: Centers for Disease Control and Prevention, National Program of Cancer Registries
(NPCR), United States Cancer Statistics (USCS) Top Ten Cancers 2011 Top Ten Cancers.
Retrieved from: http://apps.nccd.cdc.gov/uscs/toptencancers.aspx

Analysis

Table 14.1 shows a comprehensive overview of top ten cancer
sites among U.S. women of all races, as well as of white and Asian/
Pacific Islander women, from 2006 to 2010.

Interestingly, in the data for all races, the cervix does not appear at all in the top ten cancer sites list. It also does not appear in the data for white and Asian/Pacific Islander women, although other gynecological sites, such as the ovaries and uterus, do appear. This supports the fact that cervical cancer is much less common and less terminal than other cancers—especially other gynecological cancers.

Data

Table 14.2 Incidence Rate of Top Ten Cancer Sites in Black, American Indian/Alaska Native, and Hispanic Women in the United States, 2006–2010

Cancer site	Rate
Black	
1. Female breast	118.3
2. Lung and bronchus	51.0
3. Colon and rectum	46.6
4. Corpus and uterus	22.9
5. Pancreas	13.9
6. Kidney and renal pelvis	12.2
7. Non-Hodgkin lymphoma	11.7
8. Thyroid	11.2
9. Cervix	**10.3**
10. Myeloma	10.1
American Indian/Alaska Native	
1. Female breast	65.8
2. Lung and bronchus	38.2
3. Colon and rectum	29.4
4. Corpus and uterus	15.6
5. Kidney and renal pelvis	11.5
6. Non-Hodgkin lymphoma	10.2
7. Ovary	8.6
8. Thyroid	8.6
9. Pancreas	7.4
10. Cervix	**6.6**
Hispanic	
1. Female breast	90.9
2. Colon and rectum	32.6
3. Lung and bronchus	26.7
4. Corpus and uterus	20.0
5. Thyroid	17.4

(Continued)

Table 14.2 Incidence Rate of Top Ten Cancer Sites in Black, American Indian/Alaska Native, and Hispanic Women in the United States, 2006–2010 (*Continued*)

Cancer site	Rate
6. Non-Hodgkin lymphoma	15.2
7. Kidney and renal pelvis	11.4
8. Cervix	**10.9**
9. Ovary	10.9
10. Pancreas	10.2

Note: Rates are per 100,000 women and are age-adjusted to the 2000 United States standard population.

Source: Centers for Disease Control and Prevention, National Program of Cancer Registries (NPCR), United States Cancer Statistics (USCS) Top Ten Cancers 2011 Top Ten Cancers. Retrieved from: http://apps.nccd.cdc.gov/uscs/toptencancers.aspx

Analysis

Table 14.2 is an extension of data of the top ten cancer sites for black, American Indian/Native Alaskan, and Hispanic women from 2006 to 2010.

Unlike data for all races, as well as for white and Asian/Pacific Islander women, the cervix does appear as a top ten cancer site for black, American Indian/Alaska native, and Hispanic women. For black women, it is the ninth most common cancer site with a rate of 10.3. For American Indian/Alaska native women, it is tenth with a rate of 6.6. Finally, for Hispanic women, it is eighth with a rate of 10.9 (the highest rate among the three groups).

Even though the cervix does make these three lists of data, it is always in the bottom half of cancer sites—specifically, in one of the last three places. In each instance, it maintains a staggeringly lower rate compared to the other cancer sites featured on the lists.

DISCUSSION QUESTIONS

1. Cervical cancer is one of the most preventable gynecological cancers. Why do you think cervical cancer is more preventable than ovarian, uterine, and vaginal cancers?
2. According to Table 14.2, the cervix is one of the top ten cancer sites in black, American Indian/Alaska native, and Hispanic women. What might differentiate these groups from groups of white and Asian/Pacific Islander women, who do not feature cervical cancer on their lists of top ten cancers at all?

3. Some women and young girls opt to receive human papillomavirus vaccines. How can getting vaccinated for human papillomavirus help or hurt the fight against cervical cancer?
4. Two of the risk factors associated with cervical cancer are using contraceptives and smoking cigarettes. Why are women who participate in these activities more at risk for contracting the disease than women who do not?
5. Cancer cells originating in the cervix have the potential to spread to other areas of the body. Keeping in mind the female anatomy, particularly the reproductive system, what surrounding areas are cancer cells in the cervix most likely to attack?

15

CESAREAN BIRTHS

INTRODUCTION

Understanding Cesarean Births

A cesarean delivery, also frequently referred to as a C-section, is a surgical procedure commonly used to deliver a baby. Instead of a natural birth where the baby passes through the vagina, C-sections deliver the baby by taking it out through the mother's abdomen.

A female will experience three stages of labor, which can begin weeks before the actual delivery of the baby. The first stage of labor occurs when a female's contractions begin and continues until the cervix has stretched for delivery to ten centimeters. The second stage occurs when the female begins to push downward, with the cervix dilating fully and the actual delivery being made. The third stage, also known as the placental stage, begins with the birth of the baby and ends with the completed delivery of the placenta. The signs of labor and duration of each stage vary by each individual. Signs of labor may include lightening, which is when the baby moves lower in the uterus away from the rib cage to the pelvic area, or an increase in vaginal discharge, which can be clear, pink, or slightly bloody.

Unless medically necessary, a female should wait until 39 weeks to deliver a baby. If there are medical reasons for having a cesarean delivery, the C-section can be scheduled. Cesarean sections are typically safe for both the mother and the baby; however, it is a major surgery that carries risks. Recovering from a C-section also takes longer than recovering from natural, vaginal birth. C-sections may affect later attempts at vaginal births, as the incision can weaken the wall of the uterus even after healing. Infants who are delivered by C-section may also be at a higher risk of breathing problems. Other risks associated with cesarean deliveries include infection, blood loss, formation of blood clots in the legs, pelvic organs or lungs, injury to the bowel or bladder, and reaction to the medication or anesthesia that is used.

Procedure

Before a cesarean delivery, females will receive an IV to make sure they have the proper amount of fluids and medicine needed to perform the surgery. Females who undergo a cesarean delivery may be given medication with an epidural block, a spinal block, or general anesthesia to prevent pain. An epidural block numbs the lower part of the body by injecting the spine with medication, similar to a spinal block which injects the medication directly in to the spinal fluid. General anesthesia is typically used for emergency C-sections and puts the female asleep completely. A catheter is then inserted into the bladder to allow the mother to urinate during and after the surgery. A female's blood pressure, heart rate, heart rhythm, and blood oxygen level are closely monitored throughout the entire surgery.

To perform the cesarean delivery, incisions are made in the mother's abdomen and uterus. Typically, the incision line is made horizontally across the lower abdomen, just above the pubic hair line; however, in emergency cesarean deliveries, the incision may be made vertically from the navel down to the pubic area. Females may experience a feeling of pressure or pulling as the baby is delivered. After delivering the baby, the placenta is removed and the uterus and abdomen are closed with dissolvable stitches or staples.

Risk Factors

Certain females require medically necessary cesarean deliveries. C-sections are commonly performed when a female is carrying more than one baby. Specifically, if a female is carrying more than two babies, their chances of preterm labor increase, which could lead to delivery complications or fetal distress. Also, the more cesarean deliveries that a female has, the greater the risk for complications during future pregnancies such as problems with the placenta, rupturing the uterus, or hemorrhaging which would require a C-section.

Females with chronic health conditions such as high blood pressure or heart disease that require treatment during delivery may require a cesarean delivery. Additionally, females with conditions such as gestational diabetes are at an increased risk of requiring a cesarean delivery because their babies tend to be larger in size, especially if their blood sugar levels are not well controlled. The larger size of the baby increases the risk of certain complications, such as shoulder dystocia, which is when an infant's head is delivered through the vagina but the shoulders will not pass through. Females with infections such as HIV or herpes are also at a higher risk of requiring a cesarean delivery in order to prevent transmitting the virus to the infant.

Diagnosis

Medical professionals should be contacted if any of the following signs are experienced during the stages of labor: contractions every ten minutes or more often, change in color of vaginal discharge, pelvic pressure, lower backache, vaginal bleeding, or abdominal cramps with or without diarrhea.

The majority of C-sections are performed when an unexpected problem arises during delivery, including the presence of heart problems in the mother; the positioning of the baby, such as a breech presentation where the infant is upside down and the feet would be delivered first; not enough room for the baby to pass through the vagina or the fetus is too large; or signs of distress in the baby, such as problems with the umbilical cord or an abnormal heart rate. Additional complications that can require a C-section include the cervix not dilating normally or problems with the placenta. If the placenta is not formed correctly, functioning correctly, or positioned correctly in the uterus, complications such as vaginal bleeding or deprivation of oxygen and nutrients for the baby could occur.

Recovery

While most females go home three to five days after a C-section, cesarean deliveries typically require a recovery period of four to six weeks. At the end of this period, medical professionals should be contacted to ensure proper healing of the abdomen, vagina, cervix, and uterus. Discomfort and fatigue are common during this period; however, there are several ways to promote healing. Females who have undergone a C-section should rest when possible and avoid lifting anything heavier than their baby; use good posture to support the abdomen, especially during sudden movements that could affect the incision such as coughing, sneezing, or laughing; take pain medications as needed; and drink fluids to prevent constipation and replace fluids lost during delivery and breastfeeding.

During the recovery period, females may experience vaginal discharge that is initially heavy and red, but diminishes and becomes yellow or white. Afterpains are also common, similar to contractions felt during labor or menstrual cramps. Afterpains are a necessary process that helps prevent excessive bleeding by compressing the blood vessels in the uterus. Decreased hormone levels after pregnancy may also lead to hair loss and skin changes, such as the lightening of dark patches that appeared during pregnancy or the fading of stretch marks. The body will also change by losing weight from excision of the baby, placenta, and amniotic fluid. Mood changes such as irritability, anxiety, or mild depression may occur as well. Mild depression is common and typically subsides within two weeks after delivery; however, females should be aware of lasting signs or symptoms that may indicate postpartum depression.

Females can begin breastfeeding almost immediately after a cesarean delivery; however, their breasts may be sore for several days after the C-section. Engorgement, or the firming and swelling of the breasts, may be relieved by nursing the baby, using a breast pump, or applying ice packs. Breasts may also leak between feedings.

Additionally, females should routinely check their incision after a cesarean delivery. Medical professionals should be contacted if the incision is painful, red, swollen, or leaking discharge, or if a female has a fever over 100.4 degrees Fahrenheit.

DATA AND ANALYSES

Data

Table 15.1 Cesarean Delivery at 38 and 39 Weeks of Gestation, by Age of Mother: United States, 2009 and 2011

Age	38 weeks gestation in 2009	38 weeks gestation in 2011	39 weeks gestation in 2009	39 weeks gestation in 2011
Under 25	26.5	24.7	26.2	26.5
25–34 years	34.9	32.9	33.3	34.7
35 and older	45.2	42.9	42.8	44.1

Source: Martin, J.A., & Osterman, M.J.K. 2013. "Changes in cesarean delivery rates by gestational age: United States, 1996–2011." Centers for Disease Control and Prevention. Retrieved from: http://www.cdc.gov/nchs/data/databriefs/db124.pdf

Analysis

Table 15.1 above examines cesarean deliveries at 38 and 39 weeks of gestation by the age of the mother. Overall, cesarean delivery rates at 38 weeks of gestation declined, but increased at 39 weeks. From 2009 to 2011, all early-term cesarean delivery rates declined 4% to 32.2%, while full-term rates increased 3% to 30.1%.

Specifically examining the cesarean delivery rates at 38 weeks of gestation from all maternal age groups between 2009 and 2011, a decrease of more than 5% was presented. Contrastingly, cesarean delivery rates at 39 weeks of gestation increased by at least 1% for all maternal age groups.

Mothers aged 35 years and older presented the most cesarean delivery rates, followed by 25–34-year-olds, and mothers under age 25.

Data

Table 15.2 Percent Change in Cesarean Delivery Rates at 38 and 39 Weeks of Gestation by Race: United States, 2009–2011

Race	Percent change at 38 weeks gestation	Percent change at 39 weeks gestation
Non-Hispanic white	−5.8%	+2.8%
Non-Hispanic black	−4.4%	+3.8%
Hispanic	−4.8%	+6.1%
Average total	−5.3%	+4.0%

Source: Martin, J.A., & Osterman, M.J.K. 2013. "Changes in cesarean delivery rates by gestational age: United States, 1996–2011." Centers for Disease Control and Prevention. Retrieved from: http://www.cdc.gov/nchs/data/databriefs/db124.pdf

Analysis

Table 15.2 further examines the change in cesarean delivery rates at 38-weeks' gestation and 39-weeks' gestation between the years 2009 and 2011 by race. Overall, delivery rates at 38-weeks' gestation declined, while rates at 39-weeks' gestation presented an increase.

For each of the largest racial and ethnic groups, cesarean delivery rates declined at 38-weeks' gestation, with non-Hispanic white mothers presenting almost a 6% decrease to 32.2%. For non-Hispanic black mothers, over a 4% decrease to 32.4% was presented, while Hispanic mothers showed nearly a 5% decrease to 31.7%. Contrastingly, cesarean delivery rates for 39 weeks rose for each group, with Hispanic mothers presenting the greatest increase. Hispanic mothers presented over a 6% increase to 33.1%, followed by non-Hispanic black mothers, whose rates increased nearly 4% to 35.3%, and non-Hispanic white mothers, whose rates increased nearly 3% to 33.5%.

DISCUSSION QUESTIONS

1. Why did cesarean delivery rates decrease from 2009 to 2011 for 38 weeks of gestation, but increase for 39 weeks of gestation? Are more females choosing cesarean deliveries once they have reached the healthy, full-term 39 weeks of gestation?
2. Why do cesarean delivery rates increase directly with age?
3. Why do Hispanic mothers present the greatest increase in cesarean deliveries at 39 weeks of gestation? Are the cesarean deliveries medically necessary?
4. Should all nonmedically required cesarean deliveries be decreased?
5. How common are complications with cesarean deliveries? How can the recovery period of cesarean deliveries be sped up and more similar to natural, vaginal births?

16

CHILDHOOD OBESITY

INTRODUCTION

Understanding Childhood Obesity

Obesity has been at the center of health discussions for many years. Having a few extra pounds is not a cause for concern, as this rarely results in noticeable health challenges for an individual. It is when those pounds begin to interfere with one's overall health and well-being that it becomes a problem.

Obesity is a weight-based disease characterized by having such an excess amount of body fat that it poses a danger to the proper functioning of one's major organ systems, as well as the comfortable execution of one's daily activities. Obesity is not to be confused with being overweight, which means having an excess amount of body weight.

Although obesity is typically associated with adults, it is by no means exclusive to older people. Obesity can and often does also affect children. The concept of having too much body fat translates directly from adults to smaller and younger children, but diagnosis, causes, symptoms, treatment, and data are slightly different and unique for either group. In most cases, childhood obesity can actually be more dangerous than adult obesity. In fact, childhood obesity has steadily grown to become one of the most serious health problems around the world since the turn of the century. In today's United States alone, 1 in every 6 children suffers from obesity at a very young age.

Causes

Because childhood obesity is brought about by a combination of factors and does not happen instantly, it is difficult to pinpoint its exact causes. Usually, however, obesity can be linked to children's eating habits, amount of physical activity, and amount of media exposure. When children become accustomed to consuming foods and drinks that are high in sugar and calories, or are subject to environments where they cannot remain active, they begin to gain weight and body fat rapidly. The tremendous amount of advertising for fast food and unhealthy foods that children are exposed to on a daily basis through media platforms like the television, Internet, billboards, and magazines contributes to their validation of eating these foods. Moreover, unhealthy foods that are quickly made or bought and that are relatively cheap to obtain might be a more convenient choice for parents who are looking to save time and money.

Lack of breastfeeding or not following through with breastfeeding until a child reaches the age of 6 months has been cited as a cause in some cases of childhood obesity.

Although several studies have indicated that genes might play a role in the occurrence of obesity in children, more hypotheses have emerged than hard evidence. Typically, however, children of obese parents are more likely to be obese themselves.

Diagnosis

Child obesity is considerably easier to diagnose than other conditions or diseases. Since obesity deals with weight, the most obvious indication is typically physical—simply seeing an extreme amount of body fat on a child compared to the average amount of body fat on a child that is the same age and height. Moreover, there is an instant measure to test whether or not a child might be obese called the body mass index (BMI). This measurement takes into account a child's weight, height, age, and sex to calculate a number and percentile to show what weight range he or she falls into. In general, anything equal to or greater than the 95th percentile indicates obesity. BMI is especially important when parents or doctors are unsure of whether a child is overweight or obese.

Although BMI is the best way to indirectly measure body fat, there are several symptoms that are indicative of childhood obesity if they persist on a daily basis. These symptoms include:

- Constant breathlessness
- Increased sweating without much physical exertion
- Pain in the back and joints
- Inability to do physical activity for long periods of time
- Fatigue
- Difficulty falling or staying asleep

Health Risks

What makes childhood obesity so dangerous is that it is an ongoing problem that extends well into later years of life. Not only does obesity present a variety of threatening health risks for every major organ system in the body of the obese child, especially the cardiovascular system, but it also increases the probability of other, more severe health risks when the obese child becomes an adult. With immune systems that are still in the crucial developing stage, it is more difficult for children to deal with these health risks. When children gain so much weight that it begins to negatively impact their lives physically and psychologically, they have the potential to experience:

- Diabetes
- Cardiovascular disease
- High blood pressure
- High cholesterol
- Sleep apnea
- Asthma
- Heartburn
- Liver disease
- Gallstones
- Depression
- Morbidity
- Death

It is interesting to note that the aforementioned health risks that obese children face are usually ones that nonobese people must deal with only later in life. Keeping this in mind, as an obese child grows into an adult, he or she is at risk for:

- A more severe form of obesity
- Diabetes
- Stroke
- Hypertension

- Heart disease
- Kidney disease
- Several types of cancer
- Reduced life expectancy
- Depression
- Suicidal thoughts

Treatment

Fortunately, obesity is reversible and can be treated in different ways. It is true that as children grow, every inch added to their height incrementally balances the BMI for their age and drives it back to a healthier range. Unfortunately, this may take years and may not always produce the most noticeable results. Treatment for this condition is much more complex and requires a significant amount of time and effort.

Families with obese children usually try to create a schedule of consistent physical activity, to control portions, and to shift their young boy or girl's eating habits toward healthy foods like fruits and vegetables in order to lose weight. To facilitate these lifestyle interventions and professionally monitor their obese child's progress, parents may enlist the help of a team of doctors, which might include a dietician, pediatrician, physical therapist, and even a pediatric therapist if the child has been suffering from self-esteem issues or depression because of their weight. Starting this kind of treatment as soon as possible will yield the best results and keep the obese child on the path to a healthier lifestyle.

In the most extreme cases, fat-burning prescription drugs can be prescribed by the child's pediatrician or weight loss surgery can be performed if these interventions have not been effective.

DATA AND ANALYSES

Data

Table 16.1 Percentage of Childhood Obesity Among U.S. Children Aged 2–19 Based on Sex, Race, Ethnicity, and Poverty Income Ratio, 2005–2008

	PIR >350%*	PIR <130%*
Non-Hispanic white boy	10.2%	20.7%
Non-Hispanic black boy	12.5%	18.4%
Mexican American boy	22.9%	24.0%

	PIR >350%*	PIR <130%*
Non-Hispanic white girl	10.6%	18.3%
Non-Hispanic black girl	22.6%	25.1%
Mexican American girl	21.0%	16.2%

Note: PIR denotes Poverty Income Ratio.

Source: http://www.cdc.gov/nchs/data/databriefs/db51.htm

Analysis

Table 16.1 shows the complex relationships between obesity and economic status for boy and girls of three distinct ethnicities and races: non-Hispanic whites, non-Hispanic blacks, and Mexican Americans. These factors of financial, cultural, and gender status, in conjunction with the issue of child obesity, present interesting trends and provide worthwhile insight into the disease. It is worth noting that, in the table, a poverty income ratio greater than 350% denotes a high-income household, while a poverty income ratio less than 130% indicates a low-income household.

In general, all categories, with the exception of Mexican American girls, show a higher occurrence of obesity if the child comes from a lower-income household than if the child comes from a higher-income household.

Non-Hispanic white boys present the greatest difference. This category had a 10.2% obesity estimate when taking into account boys living above the 350% poverty income ratio, compared to the 20.7% estimate with those living under the 130% poverty income ratio. This means that there is double the amount of obese non-Hispanic white boys living with low-income families than there are living in high-income families.

Data

Table 16.2 Prevalence of Childhood Obesity in the United States, 1971–2008

	2–5 years old	6–11 years old	Total
1971–1974	5.0%	4.0%	5.0%
1976–1980	5.0%	6.5%	5.5%
1988–1994	7.2%	11.3%	10.0%
1999–2000	10.3%	15.1%	13.9%
2001–2002	10.6%	16.3%	15.4%

(Continued)

Table 16.2 Prevalence of Childhood Obesity in the United States, 1971–2008 (*Continued*)

	2–5 years old	6–11 years old	Total
2003–2004	13.9%	18.8%	17.1%
2005–2006	11.0%	15.1%	15.5%
2007–2008	10.4%	19.6%	16.9%

Source: http://www.cdc.gov/nchs/data/hestat/obesity_child_07_08/obesity_child_07_08. htm#table1

Analysis

In the time span of almost four decades, the percentage of obese children in the United States increased dramatically. Numbers were low in the 1970s, but quickly entered the double digits by the turn of the century, tripling and even quadrupling in certain categories. Looking at the Table 16.2, from 1971 to 2008, children between the ages of 2 and 5 went from 5.0% to 10.4%, children between the ages of 6 and 11 climbed from 4.0% to 19.6%, and in total increased from 5.0% to 16.9%. From the first time period in the table to the most recent, this accounts for a 5.4% difference in prevalence for 2–5-year-olds, followed by a whopping 15.6% difference for 6–11-year-olds, and finally, a total difference of 11.9%.

Data

Table 16.3 Change in Prevalence of Childhood Obesity in the United States, 2008–2011

Experienced change	States
Significant increase	Colorado, Pennsylvania, Tennessee
Significant decrease	California, Florida, Georgia, Iowa, Idaho, Kansas, Massachusetts, Maryland, Michigan, Minnesota, Missouri, Mississippi, New Hampshire, New Jersey, New Mexico, New York, South Dakota, Virgin Islands, Washington
No statistically significant change	Alabama, Arkansas, Arizona, Connecticut, District of Columbia, Hawaii, Illinois, Indiana, Kentucky, Montana, North Carolina, North Dakota, Nebraska, Nevada, Ohio, Oregon, Puerto Rico, Rhode Island, Vermont, Wisconsin, West Virginia
Data unavailable	Alaska, Louisiana, Maine, Oklahoma, South Carolina, Texas, Utah, Virginia, Wyoming

Source: http://www.cdc.gov/vitalsigns/ChildhoodObesity/infographic-text.html#map

Analysis

The United States has consistently clung near the top of the list of countries with the highest number of obese children. Although childhood obesity in the United States reached an all-time high with the turn of the century, a large number of states and territories actually reported a significant decrease in childhood obesity among the youngest section of their populations from 2008 to 2010. These states, including California, Washington, Florida, and New Hampshire, came from every corner of the country. Colorado, Pennsylvania, and Tennessee were the only three states to show a significant increase in the number of children dealing with obesity during the three-year time span. However, a majority of states reported no significant increase or decrease in obesity rates whatsoever. This indicates that, despite the improvement in some areas, there is still opportunity for substantial progress to be made in others.

DISCUSSION QUESTIONS

1. Obesity has afflicted so many young children during this century, more than any other period in history, that experts say the condition has reached epidemic proportions. What aspects of twenty-first-century lifestyle have contributed to the prevalence of obesity in young populations around the world?

2. Contradicting the misconception that having more money denotes having access to and eating more food, childhood obesity was found to be more common in low- and middle-income households than it is in high-income households. How can the personal finances of a family play a role in childhood obesity? Why do you think children from high-income families are less likely to suffer from obesity?

3. Because children are impressionable by nature, parents have the opportunity to teach them important lifelong lessons, especially when it comes to health and well-being. What kind of healthy eating habits and behaviors can parents instill in their children early on as they are growing up in order to help them manage their weight and prevent childhood obesity?

4. The data presented above shows a variety of U.S. states that have shown a significant increase or decrease of childhood obesity among their youth in recent years. Do you think region or location in the United States has a direct hand with these results, or are these variables purely arbitrary?

5. Several people around the country and around the world do not know how to avoid obesity until it is too late. How can major institutions like the government and education system effectively raise awareness about issues like child obesity and disseminate helpful information about how to bring this epidemic under control?

17

CHOLESTEROL LEVELS

INTRODUCTION

Understanding Cholesterol Levels

Cholesterol, a fatty substance similar to wax, finds itself in the body's bloodstream when it is produced by the organs or converted from carbon in consumed food. Contrary to popular belief, not all cholesterol is detrimental to health. In fact, it is actually crucial to life.

Only low-density lipoproteins (LDL) cholesterol, with its potential to create a plaque buildup, clog the arteries, and cause heart disease and stroke, is harmful. High-density lipoproteins (HDL) cholesterol, on the other hand, actually helps in vitamin production, digestion, creation of cell coatings, and lowered risk of the aforementioned diseases.

To understand cholesterol levels, it is important to know that each kind of cholesterol is measured as milligrams of cholesterol per deciliter of blood. This is notated as mg/dL.

There are two extremes in cholesterol levels with which these measurements become especially useful: hypercholesterolemia and hypocholesterolemia. While hypercholesterolemia refers to abnormally high levels of cholesterol in the blood (more than 200 mg/dL), hypocholesterolemia denotes abnormally low levels of it (less than 160 mg/dL).

Either one of these conditions can increase the risk of other, more serious—often deadly—conditions, including coronary heart disease, heart attack, cardiovascular diseases, and stroke. To avoid these problems, it is important to constantly monitor LDL, HDL, and total cholesterol levels and make sure they are not too high or too low.

Risk Factors

Because there are several factors that can influence them, it is easy for cholesterol levels to become imbalanced. When it comes to having high levels of LDL cholesterol, risk factors fall into the three categories of heredity, condition, and behavior. Risk factors that make people more likely to develop high levels of LDL cholesterol and low levels of HDL cholesterol include but are not limited to:

- Growing older
- Having diabetes
- Being overweight or obese
- Eating foods high in saturated fats, trans fats, dietary cholesterol, and triglycerides
- Being a woman
- Not being physically active
- Smoking cigarettes
- Drinking alcohol
- Having a family history of high cholesterol
- Inheriting a genetic condition called familial hypercholesterolemia, which increases the level of LDL cholesterol at a young age

Diagnosis

Because both hypercholesterolemia and hypocholesterolemia lack consistent or obvious signs and symptoms, a medical professional must make an official diagnosis. The most common way to check levels of cholesterol is by taking a special kind of blood test called a lipoprotein panel, which measures total, LDL, and HDL cholesterol as well as triglyceride levels. Once the vials of blood are analyzed, the levels can be measured against healthy standards and proper treatment can be administered if necessary.

Treatment

Luckily, once a person is diagnosed with high or low cholesterol, there are no complicated procedures or surgeries they need to go through in order to fix the problem. Usually, simple lifestyle changes are enough to not only keep levels of bad LDL cholesterol down but also to gradually raise levels of good HDL cholesterol in the blood.

Doctors most commonly recommend maintaining a healthy weight by exercising, consuming foods with fiber and unsaturated fats, and avoiding foods high in saturated fats, trans fats, and carbohydrates. Abstaining from drinking alcohol and smoking cigarettes is also advised. Because these kinds of lifestyle changes act as preventative measures against—not just treatments for—imbalanced cholesterol levels, a person does not have to wait until a diagnosis is made to practice them.

In extreme cases, when a person is suffering from severely high levels of LDL cholesterol, lifestyle changes must be supplemented with prescribed medications, including:

- Statin drugs
- Bile acid sequestrants
- Niacin
- Nicotinic acid
- Fibrates

In general, oral statin drugs manipulate the liver so it slows down LDL cholesterol production and works to eliminate existing LDL cholesterol in the bloodstream, while bile acid sequestrants do the same by destroying bile acid. The B vitamin niacin and nicotinic acid work together to balance cholesterol levels in the blood. This treatment is so potent that patients typically require medical supervision. Finally, fibrates target HDL levels to increase them.

DATA AND ANALYSES

Data

Table 17.1 Various Levels and Categories of Total, LDL, and HDL Cholesterol in Adults, 2012

Total cholesterol level	Total cholesterol category
Less than 200 mg/dL	Desirable
200–239 mg/dL	Borderline high
240 mg/dL and higher	High

(Continued)

Table 17.1 Various Levels and Categories of total, LDL, and HDL Cholesterol in Adults, 2012 (*Continued*)

Total cholesterol level	Total cholesterol category
LDL cholesterol level	**LDL cholesterol category**
Less than 100 mg/dL	Optimal
100–129 mg/dL	Near/above optimal
130–159 mg/dL	Borderline high
160–189 mg/dL	High
190 mg/dL and higher	Very high
HDL cholesterol level	**HDL cholesterol category**
Less than 40 mg/dL	Major risk factor for heart disease
40–59 mg/dL	The higher, the better
60 mg/dL and higher	Protective against heart disease

Source: U.S. Department of Health and Human Services, National Heart, Lung & Blood Institute, How Is High Blood Cholesterol Diagnosed? Retrieved from: https://www.nhlbi.nih.gov/health/health-topics/topics/hbc/diagnosis.html

Analysis

Table 17.1 lists the cholesterol levels that are ideal for adults to stay healthy. While levels of LDL should be less than 100mg/dL to be considered optimal, levels of HDL should be higher than 40mg/dL or they become a risk factor for heart disease. Keeping this in mind, total cholesterol levels should not exceed 200mg/dL. It is important for adults to use these guidelines to find a healthy balance of "good" and "bad" cholesterol while staying within the limits of desirable total cholesterol levels.

Data

Table 17.2 Percentage of Risk Reduction of Selected Outcomes in United States Adults Through Various Treatment Methods, 2012

Outcomes	Magnitude of risk reduction		
	Using statins per 39 mg/dL of LDL-C	Healthy dietary patterns	Physical activity
Major coronary event	21–27%	24–30%	14–20%
Any stroke	11–20%	13–29%	12–30%
Vascular mortality	9–16%	28–37%	30–40%

Source: Centers for Disease Control and Prevention, Prevention, Treatment, and Control of High Cholesterol. Retrieved from: http://www.cdc.gov/primarycare/materials/highcholesterol/index.html

Analysis

Table 17.2 shows three different methods of lowering high levels of cholesterol—using statins, maintaining a nutritious diet, and engaging in physical activity—and their percentages of risk reduction for major coronary events, strokes, and vascular mortality.

All three treatments show significant risk reduction for each outcome category. A healthy dietary pattern maintains the highest risk reduction for major coronary events and strokes (24–30% and 13–29%, respectively), while physical activity has the highest risk reduction percentage (30–40%) for vascular mortality. The risk reduction percentages would likely be even higher if the prescribed statin medication and lifestyle changes were used as treatment for any given patient at the same time.

Data

Table 17.3 Percentage of Men and Women in the United States Aged 20 and Over With High Levels of Total Cholesterol, 2009 to 2012

Age group	Men	Women
20 to 34 years old	6.0%	5.7%
35 to 44 years old	15.8%	10.4%
45 to 54 years old	18.0%	18.7%
55 to 64 years old	14.1%	26.6%
65 to 74 years old	8.1%	19.6%
75 years and older	5.5%	16.2%

Note: All data is age-adjusted and considers levels of total cholesterol greater than or equal to 240 mg/dL.

Source: http://www.cdc.gov/nchs/data/hus/2012/065.pdf

Analysis

Table 17.3 shows the relationship between high cholesterol levels, age, and gender. In general, the percentage of men and women with high cholesterol increased until the 55–64 age range. At this point, it began to reverse its trend and slowly decrease.

From the 45–54 age range on, the women's percentages grew significantly compared to that of the men. In some cases, the numbers even tripled. This supports the fact that women are more likely to have higher cholesterol levels than men.

DISCUSSION QUESTIONS

1. Cholesterol is a substance that humans can consume and that can be considered good or bad. Can you think of any other substances that are simultaneously good in moderation and bad in excess?
2. To lower LDL cholesterol levels, doctors recommend maintaining a nutritious diet of foods high in fiber. What are some foods that meet this criterion?
3. Table 17.2 shows the benefits of healthy dietary patterns and physical activity in relation to cholesterol levels. With what other conditions or health issues might a regimen of healthy food and exercise be good treatment or preventative measure?
4. The standard desirable level of HDL cholesterol, which is considered the "good" cholesterol, is less than 40 mg/dL. What effect do you think an excess of HDL cholesterol in the bloodstream might have on the human body?
5. Older people are much more likely to contract hypercholesterolemia than younger people are. What are some possible reasons why older age plays such a major role in the likelihood of suffering from health problems related to cholesterol?

18

COLON/RECTAL CANCER

INTRODUCTION

Understanding Colon/Rectal Cancer

Two major actors of the human digestive system are the colon and rectum. The colon, which is also known as the large intestine, is responsible for processing waste into the connected rectum, which then stores the processed waste until the body is ready to dispose of it. The colon and rectum are as important to the body as they are susceptible to polyps, or abnormal growths, that have the ability to turn cancerous.

Colon and rectal cancer usually occur together because the two affected organs are attached and constantly working together. Because of this proximity, *colorectal cancer* is commonly used to refer to the afflicted area. When cancer overtakes the colon and rectum, it can be devastating to the digestive system if left untreated.

Symptoms

In many cases, people can live with colorectal cancer for years before noticing any related symptoms. Although colorectal cancer warning signs are uncommon during the cancer's early stages, they do become more apparent in its later stages. The most common symptoms for colorectal cancer include:

- Changes in bowel movements
- Blood in or on stool

- Long, thin stool
- Constipation
- Persistent diarrhea
- Rectal cramping
- Stomach pains and aches
- Sudden, inexplicable weight loss
- Bloating
- Loss of appetite

Diagnosis

Doctors recommend yearly screening tests that check for polyps in the colon or rectum and that help patients monitor those polyps in case they turn into colorectal cancer. These screening tests also have the ability to diagnose colorectal cancer if the polyps have already become cancerous, but are usually conducted when no symptoms are present. Aside from screening tests, there are also several diagnostic tests that can detect colorectal cancer once a person displays related symptoms.

Screening and diagnostic tests are essentially the same. The most common forms of these tests are the high-sensitivity fecal occult blood test, colonoscopy, and CT scans. A fecal blood test involves sending in samples of stool to an office or laboratory where a doctor looks for visible or invisible traces of blood. A colonoscopy takes a look at the colon and rectum from inside the body, while CT scans and other medical imaging technologies does the same from outside of the body.

Risk Factors

Colorectal cancer is like most other cancers in that its risk factors generally span the realm of lifestyle choices, genetics, and family history, among other aspects. Keeping this in mind, the main risk factors for colorectal cancer include:

- Having inflammatory bowel disease
- Having Crohn's disease
- Having ulcerative colitis
- Having a family history of colorectal cancer or polyps
- Having genetic syndromes like familial adenomatous polyposis or Lynch syndrome
- Lacking physical activity

- Eating a diet low in fiber, high in fat, or with few vegetables or fruits
- Excessively drinking alcohol
- Using tobacco
- Being overweight or obese

While there are several risk factors for colorectal cancer, there are many preventative measures to combat or reverse them. Doctors normally advise candidates for colorectal cancer, whether or not uncontrollable risk factors like age and genetics apply to them, to increase physical activity, eat more fruits and vegetables, eat less foods that are high in animal fats, and avoid substances like alcohol or tobacco.

Treatment

Colorectal cancer is much easier to cure when it is found in its early stages. In fact, according to the Centers for Disease Control and Prevention, about nine out of ten people whose case of colorectal cancer is detected early and treated are still alive five years later. In these cases, the cancerous polyps are usually removed through surgery. However, chemotherapy and radiation are other options that can be recommended by doctors or other medical professionals treating the afflicted patient.

When colorectal cancer has advanced to later stages and possibly even spread to other organs, it becomes more difficult to cure. People still have the option of surgery, chemotherapy, and radiation, but the treatment ultimately used depends largely on the stage of the cancer. Surgery cannot be performed if the cancer has affected surrounding organs. It is also worth noting that once polyps are removed and the colon cannot be attached back to the rectum, a permanent colostomy may be performed.

DATA AND ANALYSES

Data

Table 18.1 Rate of Three Most Common Cancers and Leading Causes of Cancer Death Among Men, 2013

Three most common cancers	
Prostate cancer	126.1
Lung cancer	74.1
Colorectal cancer	46.4

(Continued)

Table 18.1 Rate of Three Most Common Cancers and Leading Causes of Cancer Death Among Men, 2013 (*Continued*)

Three leading causes of cancer death	
Lung cancer	60.1
Prostate cancer	21.8
Colorectal cancer	18.7

Note: All rates in table are per 100,000 men of all races and Hispanic origins combined in the United States.

Source: Centers for Disease Control and Prevention, Cancer among Men. Retrieved from: http://www.cdc.gov/cancer/dcpc/data/men.htm

Analysis

Table 18.1 shows colorectal cancer's effect on men in the United States in 2013. Coincidentally, colorectal cancer ranked third on both lists of most common cancers and the leading causes of cancer death, with rates of 46.4 and 18.7, respectively. It ranked behind prostate and lung cancers in both instances. Even though its rate is either two or three times that of the top cancer, the data shows that colorectal cancer remains a formidable health threat to men in the United States.

Data

Table 18.2 Rate of Three Most Common Cancers and Leading Causes of Cancer Death Among Women, 2013

Three most common cancers	
Breast cancer	118.7
Lung cancer	52.4
Colorectal cancer	35.4
Three leading causes of cancer death	
Lung cancer	37.9
Breast cancer	21.9
Colorectal cancer	13.0

Note: All rates in table are per 100,000 women of all races and Hispanic origins combined in the United States.

Source: Centers for Disease Control and Prevention, Cancer among Women. Retrieved from: http://www.cdc.gov/cancer/dcpc/data/women.htm

Analysis

Table 18.2 shows colorectal cancer's effect on women in the United States in 2013. As for men, colorectal cancer ranked third on both lists of most common cancers and the leading causes of cancer death, with rates of 35.4 and 13.0, respectively. It ranked behind breast and lung cancers in both instances. The data in numbers between U.S. men and women are strikingly similar, which seems to suggest that gender does not play a significant role in colorectal cancer contraction and death rates.

Data

Table 18.3 Colorectal Cancer Death Rates by Age in People of All Races in the United States, 2010

Age	Death rate
<1 year old	Data not available
1–19 years old	Data not available
20–24 years old	0.2
25–29 years old	0.5
30–34 years old	1.0
35–39 years old	2.1
40–44 years old	4.2
45–49 years old	8.0
50–54 years old	13.8
55–59 years old	20.4
60–64 years old	30.8
65–69 years old	43.9
70–74 years old	62.8
75–79 years old	89.3
80–84 years old	125.6
>85 years old	199.5

Note: All rates in table are per 100,000 people in the United States.

Source: http://apps.nccd.cdc.gov/uscs/cancersbyageandrace.aspx?Gender=Male&Count=false&Population=false&DataType=Mortality&RateType=AgeadjType&CancerSite=Colon%20and%20Rectum&Year=2010&Site=Colon%20and%20Rectum&SurveyInstanceID=1

Analysis

Table 18.3 shows the rate of colorectal cancer death rates by the age of all races in the United States in 2010. Although data is not available for children in the <1–19-year-old age group (most likely because the colorectal cancer death rate is simply not as significant as other cancer death rates), the remainder of the data shows an interesting trend that supports the fact that increasing age is a key risk factor for colorectal cancer. In general, the older the age group, the higher the rate of colorectal cancer death in 2010. For instance, the 20–24 age group had a 0.2 death rate, while the older-than-85 age group had a 199.5 death rate.

DISCUSSION QUESTIONS

1. Colorectal cancer is easier to cure when detected early. What are other cancers that share this characteristic, and what are some reasons why early cancer detection is key to proper, potentially game-changing treatment?

2. One of the main risk factors for colorectal cancer is eating a diet that is high in animal fats and low in fiber. Why might this pattern of consumption be harmful or carcinogenic for organs like the colon and rectum?

3. Fecal blood tests, colonoscopies, and CT scans are all types of screening and diagnostic tests, but whether they are dubbed screening or diagnostic depends on one factor. What is the main difference between these two forms of tests?

4. Like other cancers, colorectal cancer has the potential to spread to surrounding organs and tissue. Using your knowledge of the human body and its organ systems, which organs near the colon and rectum would be most at risk?

5. Polyps in the body are abnormal growths that may or may not eventually turn into cancerous growths. How might these kinds of abnormal growths form in the colon or rectum, and what makes the polyps become cancerous?

19

CONGENITAL DEFECTS

INTRODUCTION

A congenital defect is a serious condition that results in changes in one or more parts of a newborn's body. Birth defects can impact almost any part of the body, including the baby's heart, brain, limbs, etc. Birth defects can have effects on how the body functions, how it looks or both. The severity of birth defects can vary considerably from individual to individual. Depending on the nature of the defect, the types of diagnostic tests undertaken and other factors, birth defects may be detected in utero, at birth, or any time after birth. The majority of birth defects are detected during the first year of life. The prognosis of a birth defect will depend on a number of factors, including the nature of the birth defect, its severity, and the treatment options made available to the individual. Birth defects are one of the leading causes of infant deaths, accounting for more than 20% of all infant deaths. Unfortunately, birth defects are also relatively common, affecting approximately 1 in every 33 babies born each year in the United States.

Prevention

Birth defects can develop during any stage of pregnancy. Most defects develop during the first trimester when the major organs of the fetus are under development. However, it is also possible for defects to occur later in development. While not all birth defects can be prevented, there are steps that women can take both before and during pregnancy to reduce the likelihood that their baby will suffer from a birth defect. To reduce the risks of congenital defects, all women who are pregnant or who are planning to become pregnant should adopt the following risk prevention strategies:

Women should take 400 micrograms of folic acid every day. Folic acid, a B vitamin, can help prevent major birth defects of the baby's brain and spine, such as anencephaly and spina bifida. By consuming adequate amounts of folic acid, women can help reduce the risk that their baby will suffer from one of these very serious ailments.

Women should avoid all alcohol throughout the entire pregnancy. When a pregnant woman consumes alcohol, alcohol passes to the baby through the placenta. Alcohol can have a number of adverse effects on the fetus, including fetal alcohol spectrum disorder. Accordingly, pregnant women are strongly advises to avoid all alcohol consumption.

Pregnant women should not smoke and should avoid exposure to secondhand smoke. Smoking during pregnancy poses a number of potential risks to the fetus, including premature birth, certain birth defects (including cleft palate) and infant death. Even exposure to secondhand smoke carries these risks.

Avoid the use of illegal drugs and limit the use of other medications. Illegal or "street" drugs can lead to a number of very serious birth defects and even death and, as such, should not be used at all during pregnancy. Even prescription drugs can be harmful to a fetus. Women who are pregnant or are trying to become pregnant should discuss all medications, including prescription medications, vitamins, over-the-counter drugs and herbal medicines, with their health care provider.

Prevent infections. Certain infections acquired by a pregnant mother can result in birth defects or otherwise cause harm to the unborn baby. As such, pregnant women should be extra careful to stay healthy during their pregnancy and to limit exposure to potentially infectious agents.

Maintain a healthy weight. Women who are obese, meaning those who have a body mass index (BMI) of 30 or higher before pregnancy, are at a higher risk for complications during pregnancy. Maternal obesity also increases the risks that the mother will give birth to a child with birth defects. Women are advised to reach a healthy weight before attempting to become pregnant.

Have regular office visits with one's medical provider. While not all birth defects can be prevented, proper health care before and during pregnancy may increase the likelihood of a positive outcome for the mother and the baby. For some birth defects, early detection may facilitate effective treatment.

DATA AND ANALYSES

Data

Table 19.1 National Estimates for 21 Selected Major Birth Defects, 2004–2006

Birth defects*	Cases per births	Estimated annual number of cases
Adjusted for maternal race/ethnicity**		
Central nervous system defects		
Anencephaly	1 in 4,859	859
Spina bifida without anencephaly	1 in 2,858	1,460
Encephalocele	1 in 12,235	341
Eye defects		
Anophthalmia/microphthalmia	1 in 5,349	780
Cardiovascular defects		
Common truncus	1 in 13,876	301
Transposition of great arteries	1 in 3,333	1,252
Tetralogy of Fallot	1 in 2,518	1,657
Atrioventricular septal defect	1 in 2,122	1,966
Hypoplastic left heart syndrome	1 in 4,344	960
Orofacial defects		
Cleft palate without cleft lip	1 in 1,574	2,651
Cleft lip with or without cleft palate	1 in 940	4,437
Gastrointestinal defects		
Esophageal atresia/tracheoesophageal fistula	1 in 4,608	905
Rectal and large intestinal atresia/stenosis	1 in 2,138	1,952
Musculoskeletal defects		
Reduction deformity, upper limbs	1 in 2,869	1,454
Reduction deformity, lower limbs	1 in 5,949	701
Gastroschisis	1 in 2,229	1,871
Omphalocele	1 in 5,386	775
Diaphragmatic hernia	1 in 3,836	1,088

(Continued)

Table 19.1 National Estimates for 21 Selected Major Birth Defects, 2004–2006 (*Continued*)

Birth defects*	Cases per births	Estimated annual number of cases
Adjusted for maternal age**		
Chromosomal anomalies		
Trisomy 13	1 in 7,906	528
Trisomy 21 (Down syndrome)	1 in 691	6,037
Trisomy 18	1 in 3,762	1,109

* The national estimates data come from 14 birth defects surveillance programs: Arkansas, Arizona, California [8-county Central Valley], Colorado, Georgia [5-county metropolitan Atlanta], Illinois, Iowa, Kentucky, Massachusetts, North Carolina, Oklahoma, Puerto Rico, Texas, and Utah. The number of live births represented by these 14 programs from 2004–2006 was 4,038,506.

** For this study, researchers took into account maternal age (for Trisomy 13, 21, and 18) and maternal race/ethnicity, which allows state and local programs to use these estimates as a point of reference for comparison with future prevalence estimates. Adjustments are based on the United States live birth population, 2004–2006.

Source: Centers for Disease Control and Prevention, Birth Defects. Retrieved from: http://www.cdc.gov/ncbddd/birthdefects/data.html

Analysis

Table 19.1 shows the number of cases per birth and the estimated number of cases for 21 selected major birth defects. While not all birth defects can be prevented, it is clear that deficiencies in folic acid can lead to the development of major birth defects of the baby's brain and spine, such as anencephaly and spina bifida. Nonetheless, there continue to be nearly 2,500 cases of anencephaly and spina bifida. Based on this finding, it would appear that continued education about the importance of folic acid is necessary as are efforts to increase the availability of folic acid supplements to pregnant women.

The data also shows that Trisomy 21, or Down syndrome is the birth defect that occurs most frequently. Down syndrome occurs when an individual has a full or partial extra copy of chromosome 21. Individuals with Down syndrome typically experience intellectual disability, characteristic facial appearances, and weak muscle tone. They may also experience a variety of other birth defects, including heart defects and digestive abnormalities. There is no cure for Down syndrome but there may be treatments for the birth defects that often accompany the disorder.

Data

Table 19.2 Racial/ethnic Differences in the Occurrence of Birth Defects

Compared with infants of non-Hispanic white mothers			
Infants of non-Hispanic black or African American mothers had		**Infants of Hispanic mothers had**	
Higher birth prevalence of these birth defects:	Lower birth prevalence of these birth defects:	Higher birth prevalence of these birth defects:	Lower birth prevalence of these birth defects:
Tetralogy of Fallot	Cleft palate	Anencephaly	Tetralogy of Fallot
Lower limb reduction defects	Cleft lip with or without cleft palate	Spina bifida	Hypoplastic left heart syndrome
Trisomy 18	Esophageal atresia or tracheoesophageal fistula	Encephalocele	Cleft palate
	Gastroschisis	Gastroschisis	Esophageal atresia or tracheoesophageal fistula
	Down syndrome	Down syndrome	

Source: http://www.cdc.gov/ncbddd/birthdefects/data.html

Analysis

As Table 19.2 demonstrates, for certain birth defects, defects vary by racial or ethnic group. These findings can be helpful to researchers who are seeking to reduce the occurrence of birth defects. Pinpointing why some birth defects occur more or less often in certain groups may lead to the discovery of interventions that will aid in the reduction of these racial and ethnic disparities.

DISCUSSION QUESTIONS

1. There are a number of measures that pregnant women can take to reduce the likelihood that their baby will be affected by a birth defect and yet, birth defects continue to be fairly common. Do you think women receive enough information about what they can do to prevent birth defects? If not, what improvements can be made to the public information that is current available concerning birth defect prevention?
2. Advanced maternal age is a risk factor for certain birth defects. Increasingly, women are having babies at older ages. Do you think that this will lead to higher numbers of birth defects in the future or are older mothers sufficiently monitored and tested so that there is no likely to be an increase in the number of birth defects?

3. There are diagnostic tests that can determine whether a fetus has certain chromosomal anomalies. Do you think that all pregnant women should be required to undergo these tests?
4. The use of certain substances (including illicit drugs, certain prescription drugs, alcohol, and tobacco) during pregnancy has been linked with the development of birth defects. Do you believe that pregnant women who use these substances during pregnancy should face criminal prosecution?
5. Folic acid is essential for preventing certain types of birth defects. Do you believe that more foods should be fortified with folic acid to increase the likelihood that women of childbearing age will receive adequate folic acid?

20

CONTRACEPTIVE USE

INTRODUCTION

Understanding Contraceptive Use

When sexually active men or women want to delay pregnancy or avoid it altogether, they usually turn to contraceptives. Also known as birth control, contraceptives refer to any device or practice used to prevent a man's sperm from fertilizing a woman's egg. They come in various forms but, while they are highly effective, are not guaranteed to work every time a couple has sexual intercourse. It is worth noting that although most contraceptive methods are made for women, they are not exclusive to them. In fact, there are some contraceptive measures that men can take or use that are highly effective in reducing the probability of pregnancy.

Contraceptives are usually designated into two umbrella categories: reversible methods of contraception and permanent methods of contraception. As their names suggest, reversible methods can be undone, removed, or stopped immediately to reverse the contraceptive effects, while permanent methods cannot be reversed.

Reversible Methods

Reversible contraceptives are far more common than permanent contraceptives because they are easier to undo or "reverse" for sexually active users who eventually change their minds about becoming pregnant. Reversible methods of contraception fall into four subcategories, including intrauterine, hormonal, barrier, and fertility awareness-based methods. In general, intrauterine methods involve devices placed in the uterus, hormonal methods hinder ovulation and fertilization with hormones like progestin and estrogen, barrier methods physically prevent sperm from reaching the egg, and fertility awareness-based methods are unique to a woman's monthly fertility pattern. Some reversible forms of contraception include:

- Copper T intrauterine device or IUD: A T-shaped device that can be kept in the uterus for up to ten years
- Levonorgestrel intrauterine system or LNG IUD: A T-shaped device that can be kept in the uterus for up to five years and releases small amounts of progestin over time
- Implant: A rod that is placed in a woman's upper arm and releases progestin over time
- Injection: A shot of progestin in a woman's buttocks or arm that is administered every three months
- Combined oral contraceptives: A prescription pill that contains two hormones, progestin and estrogen
- Progestin pill: A prescription pill that contains only one hormone, progestin
- Patch: A prescription skin patch placed on a woman's buttocks, abdomen, or upper body for three-week intervals that releases both progestin and estrogen into the bloodstream
- Vaginal ring: A ring placed in the vagina for up to three weeks that releases progestin and estrogen
- Emergency contraception: Any intrauterine device or pill that can be taken within five days of unprotected sex to prevent fertilization
- Male condom: A waterproof, elastic cover placed on the penis that physically prevents sperm from entering a woman's body and prevents the transmission of STDs
- Female condom: A lubricated insert placed in the vagina that physically prevents sperm from entering a woman's body and prevents the transmission of STDs
- Spermicides: Any sperm-killing foam, gel, cream, or tablet that is placed in the vagina less than an hour before sexual intercourse and can be kept there for approximately six to eight hours

- Diaphragm: A cup-shaped device placed in the vagina with spermicide to cover the cervix and kill or block sperm
- Natural family planning: The practice of not engaging in sexual intercourse when a woman is fertile

Permanent Methods

Permanent methods of contraception are usually opted for by men or women who know they never want to have a baby. Permanent methods usually involve surgery that, once performed, cannot be undone. The most common permanent forms of contraception, all of which have a failure rate that is less than 1%, include:

- Female sterilization or tubal ligation: An operation that closes the fallopian tubes so that sperm cannot reach the egg
- Transcervical sterilization: An operation that inserts a tube into the fallopian tubes to plug them with scar tissue so that sperm cannot reach the egg
- Male sterilization or vasectomy: An operation that blocks the pathway of sperm travelling from the testicles to the penis

Side Effects

Because many contraceptives upset the natural functioning of the human reproductive system, mainly that of a woman, there are many side effects associated with using them. Women taking contraceptives that involve progestin and estrogen supplements tend to exhibit more side effects than women using other contraceptive methods like female condoms. Some of the most common side effects of these contraceptives include:

- Nausea
- Stomach cramps
- Discoloration of skin
- Change in appetite
- Acne
- Hair growth
- Change in menstrual flow
- Breast tenderness, enlargement, or discharge
- Vaginal discharge

Some women who use contraceptives experience side effects that are far more severe. Although these side effects are extremely rare, they can be life-threatening and act as a good indicator to stop using birth control immediately. The more severe side effects of contraceptives include:

- Speech problems
- Numbness of limbs
- Fatigue
- Dark-colored urine
- Loss of vision
- Extended menstrual bleeding
- Swelling of the limbs
- Depression

DATA AND ANALYSES

Data

Table 20.1 Typical Use Failure Rates of Reversible and Permanent Methods of Contraception in the United States, 2013

Contraceptive method	Failure rate
Copper T intrauterine device	0.8%
Levonorgestrel intrauterine system	0.2%
Implant	0.05%
Injection	6.0%
Combined oral contraceptives	9.0%
Progestin pill	9.0%
Patch	9.0%
Vaginal ring	9.0%
Diaphragm	12%
Male condom	18%
Female condom	21%
Spermicide	28%
Fertility awareness	24%
Tubal ligation	<1%
Transcervical sterilization	<1%
Vasectomy	<1%

Source: Centers for Disease Control and Prevention, Reproductive Health, Contraception. Retrieved from: http://www.cdc.gov/reproductivehealth/unintendedpregnancy/contraception.htm

Analysis

The effectiveness of all contraceptive methods is not guaranteed. Popular to contrary belief, it is possible for a woman to become pregnant while using them. Failure rates differ among the various methods of birth control, however, with some ranking higher or lower on a scale of effectiveness. In general, there is a smaller chance of failure when using permanent methods like tubal ligation, transcervical sterilization, and vasectomy (all less than 1%) than there is with reversible methods. Reversible methods that share the failure rate of these three permanent methods include copper T intrauterine devices (0.8%), levonorgestrel intrauterine systems (0.2%), and implants (0.05%). The contraceptive with the highest failure rate is spermicide (28%).

Data

Table 20.2 Percentage of U.S. Women Using Sterilization or Contraceptive Pills by Age, 2006–2010

Age	Female sterilization	Contraceptive pill
15 to 19 years	*	53%
20 to 24 years	2.6%	47%
25 to 29 years	16%	33%
30 to 34 years	30%	25%
35 to 39 years	35%	17%
40 to 44 years	51%	9.8%

* *Note*: Figure does not meet standards of reliability or precision.

Source: Jones, J., Mosher, W., Daniels, K., "Current Contraceptive Use in the United States, 2006–2010, and Changes in Patterns of Use Since 1995." National Health Statistic Report No. 60, Oct. 18, 2012. Retrieved from: http://www.cdc.gov/nchs/data/nhsr/nhsr060.pdf

Analysis

Table 20.2 compares the usage of one type of permanent contraception with that of one type of reversible contraception—sterilization and hormone-based contraceptive pills, respectively—among women of different age groups in the United States.

The 30–34 age group shows a major shift in women's contraceptive use from reversible to permanent methods. A majority of the women younger than this age group use the pill, but more women aged 30 and over opt for sterilization. There is an inverse relationship on either side of the age range. As pill consumption increases, sterilization decreases, and vice versa.

Approximately 53% of teenagers in the 15–19 age range take the pill, compared to the 9.8% of women in the 40–44 age range who take it. Although accurate data is not available for teenagers choosing sterilization, it can be inferred from the table trend that the 51% of sterilized women in the 40–44 age range is matched with a very small percentage of sterilized teenagers.

DISCUSSION QUESTIONS

1. Although there are some for men, a majority of contraceptives today are made for women to use. What kind of contraceptive that has not yet been invented do you think would be an effective way for men to prevent pregnancy?
2. According to the data above, spermicide on its own has the highest failure rate among other contraceptives. What contraceptive can spermicide be used with, and how might this have an impact on the typical use failure rate?
3. Some contraceptives are inexpensive but have a higher success rate, while others are more costly but show side effects. What do you think men and women should prioritize when deciding on what kind of contraceptive to use?
4. Birth control has existed and been used by men and women for centuries, but many of the contraceptives people know and use today emerged and became popular during the twentieth century. What are some possible reasons for this?
5. In some cases, a woman relying upon contraceptives could still experience an unintended pregnancy. With what contraceptives might a woman become pregnant, and how might this occur?

21

DEPRESSION

INTRODUCTION

Depression is a serious mental illness that is more than regular sadness. It is normal to feel sad or anxious at some points in your life, like when very stressed or grieving the loss of a loved one. In those situations, you might be depressed, but not suffering from depression, which is a mental illness.

Depression is described as a period of two or more weeks marked by sadness, hopelessness, anxiety, suicidal thoughts, and other accompanying symptoms. Many people who suffer from this also have feelings of worthlessness, so they do not seek help, believing that they are not worth the time or effort to "fix." However, with medication, psychotherapy, and other treatments, it is possible for the majority of depression sufferers to overcome their illness.

Types of Depression

There are a wide array of illnesses that can be responsible for making someone feel depressed. These include: major depression (also known as major depressive disorder), minor depression, dysthymia, and bipolar disorder.

Major depressive disorder involves a combination of debilitating symptoms that interfere with your ability to eat, sleep, enjoy activities, and function well at work or school. These tend to be epi-sodic rather than chronic, with some people experiencing one while others experience them repeatedly throughout their life.

Minor depression is referred to as having some symptoms for two or more weeks without meeting the full criteria for major depres-sion, though these sufferers are at high risk for developing major depressive disorder. Some causes of this are psychotic depression (accompanied by odd thoughts and hallucinations or delusions), postpartum depression (after pregnancy), and seasonal affective disorder (depression during winter months).

Dysthymia, or dysthymic disorder, is identified by symptoms lasting two or more years, though they may not be severe enough to interfere with your regular functions, making it harder to iden-tify. People with this disorder run a greater chance of experiencing a major depressive episode.

Bipolar disorder is characterized by episodes of both mania and depression, separating it from dysthymia and major depressive disorder. In this instance, the sufferer will have periods of severe depression (usually lasting two or more weeks), broken by periods of normal moods or manic behavior. People with bipolar disorder are also more likely to develop a psychotic disorder.

Symptoms

People suffering from depression exhibit a wide array of symp-toms, since each person handles stress and emotional disturbances differently. Some of the general indicators of depression are:

- Sleeping too much or too little
- Being unable to avoid negative thoughts no matter what you do to avoid them
- Feeling hopeless about the negative aspects of your life, as though there is nothing you can do to change them
- Losing interest in daily activities, especially those you once enjoyed, or finding it hard to concentrate on routine tasks
- Losing your appetite or now eating much more than before, especially sweets and fatty foods
- Feeling angry, irritable, or violent without an apparent cause
- Reckless behavior like driving too fast or using drugs
- Unexplainable aches and pains or a loss of energy
- Feelings of self-loathing
- Feeling suicidal

Depression in Children and Young Adults

Depression can affect any person at any time, regardless of age, so it is important to recognize the difference between adults and minors when it comes to how this illness expresses itself.

Children tend to display traits of worry, anxiety, and fear. While some display sadness and depressed children tend to be underweight, the most common and easily recognized indicators are separation anxiety and a general refusal to go to school.

Teens are more inclined to self-harm, claim they are misunderstood, get into fights, argue with parents or teachers, avoiding social interaction, doing poorly or not attending school, and having problems with drugs and alcohol.

People of all ages tend to be low energy, easily confused, have memory problems, report irritability, suffer aches and pains, and lose interest in daily activities.

Risk Factors

A number of situations and traits can make someone more inclined to suffer from depression at some point in his or her life. Having depression as a teen or child makes someone much more likely to have it as an adult, just as having an anxiety or personality disorder contributes to a greater incidence of this illness. Experiencing a traumatic event may also lead to depression, especially if you develop post-traumatic stress disorder as a result.

Chronic illnesses, such as diabetes or cancer, can make someone more likely to suffer from depression. Chronic pain also contributes to this, as do personality traits like having low self-esteem, being overly dependent on others, and being generally pessimistic.

Abusing alcohol and drugs tends to cause depression, though having a relative who abused alcohol or drugs tends to contribute to depression as well. Having blood relatives who have severe mood or psychotic disorders, such as bipolar disorder, or have committed suicide contributes to this as well.

Ways to Avoid Depression

Studies show that those who take on many tasks at once are at greater risk of depression due to stress or failure to meet the expectations they have for themselves. Staying physically healthy, exercising regularly, and staying positive are the surest ways to avoid this illness, as this ensures you maintain a good hormonal and chemical balance in your brain, preventing some causes of depression. A good diet is also important here. Avoiding alcohol and drugs is also a huge factor in avoiding depression.

Putting off extreme decisions during times of stress can help as well, as you will not need to worry about the consequences of your choices until you make them. As such, it can be good to wait until a period of calmness or low stress arrives if you need to make life-altering decisions. Do not blame yourself for negative events or outcomes, as this will amplify any tendency toward depression. Volunteering can also prevent depression by increasing feelings of self-worth, confidence, and optimism. This helps you feel grateful toward what you have, and gratitude in such things is another great way of avoiding depression.

In short, getting exercise and fresh air, being grateful for what you have, doing good deeds, and eating well are the easiest ways to ensure your disposition stays positive and well away from any signs of depression.

DATA AND ANALYSES

Data

Table 21.1 Suicides per 100,000 People by Year and Age Group

	10–24	25–64	65+
1991	9.4	15.1	19.9
1993	9.5	14.9	18.8
1995	9.2	14.8	17.8
1997	8.2	14.3	16.4
1999	7.1	13.7	15.7
2001	7.0	14.3	15.5
2003	6.9	14.8	14.9
2005	7.2	15.3	15.3
2007	6.9	15.9	14.9
2009	7.2	16.1	15.2

Source: Centers for Disease Control and Prevention, National Suicide Statistics at a Glance Trends in Suicide Rates among Both Sexes, by Age Group, United States, 1991–2009. Retrieved from: http://www.cdc.gov/violenceprevention/suicide/statistics/trends02.html

Analysis

Table 21.1 examines the rate of suicide in each major age group, focusing on the past two decades. Young adults have the lowest suicide rates, and that rate dropped significantly from 1991 to 2009.

The elderly population has a higher rate, but the decrease during this time period was even more significant, with 4.7 fewer suicides happening per 100,000 people, whereas young adults had only 2.2 fewer. Mature adults, the 25–64 range, began to drop from 1991 to1999, but increased steadily from 2001 to 2009.

Data

Table 21.2 Statistical Percentages of Depressed Persons by Group

	Percentage
Age	
12–17	4.3
18–39	4.7
40–59	7.3
60 and older	4.0
Sex	
Female	6.7
Male	4.0
Race and Hispanic Origin	
Mexican American	6.3
Non-Hispanic black	6.0
Non-Hispanic white	4.8
Total	5.4

Source: Centers for Disease Control and Prevention, Percentage of Persons 12 Years of Age and Older with Depression by Demographic Characteristics: United States, 2005–2006. Retrieved from: http://www.cdc.gov/mentalhealth/data_stats/depression-chart-txt.htm

Analysis

Table 21.2 examines the different races, ages, and sexes, breaking down which are more or less likely to suffer depression. Men are far less likely to be depressed than women. At all ages, people are diagnosed at roughly the same rate, except the 40–59 category, which shows a 2.6% increase. Mexican Americans are most likely to be depressed while non-Hispanic whites are the least.

DISCUSSION QUESTIONS

1. Depression is a very noticeable, debilitating mental condition. Why might a family member or friend not notice or recommend a depressed person seek help?

2. Chronic illnesses can lead to depression, but this is rarely talked about. Should more be done to provide these sufferers with counseling?

3. Depression can often be alleviated or prevented by the same factors relating to good health (exercise, sunlight, healthy food), yet depressed people often do not take these steps to help themselves. Should this be treated as part of the illness or as a patient's unwillingness to help his or her self?

4. A larger percentage of minorities are depressed compared to the average for the whole population. Why do you think this might be?

5. The signs and symptoms of depression in children and teens are often missed or written off, and in many cases, people who need serious help are ignored. What can be done to break these stereotypes and get such individuals the assistance they need?

22

DIABETES

INTRODUCTION

Understanding Diabetes

Diabetes is a metabolic disorder that affects the pancreas and the body's ability to produce and absorb insulin. Metabolism is the process through which our bodies break down and absorb nutrients. As a result, metabolic disorders, such as diabetes can be very damaging if not controlled. There are three types of diabetes: Type

Type 1, or insulin dependent diabetes, means the pancreas no longer makes the hormones that control blood glucose levels. The pancreas is a digestive organ found just behind the stomach that produces the hormones insulin and glucagon. When the body breaks down carbohydrates, insulin regulates the level of glucose in the blood by allowing it to enter the body's cells, leading to energy and growth. If the levels drop too low, glucagon brings them back up again by breaking down fatty tissues. People with type 1 diabetes need insulin injections and, occasionally, glucagon injections to control their glucose. They usually follow a strict diet as well, to increase their control. Roughly 10% of all diabetics suffer from this type of diabetes.

When individuals have Type 2 diabetes, their the bodies do not produce enough insulin, or the insulin is not absorbed properly. This is most commonly associated with overweight people, which is why some mistakenly call type 2 diabetes the "fat people's disease," but this isn't correct. Anyone can develop type 2 diabetes, regardless of body fat. Type 2 diabetes tends to get progressively worse until the patient needs insulin tablets.

Gestational diabetes affects pregnant women, and is usually controlled through diet and exercise. Ten to twenty percent of pregnant women will need insulin to control their glucose. Otherwise, the baby may suffer complications.

Symptoms

Diabetes can be tricky, because the symptoms for high and low blood glucose, both of which are signs of this illness, can be very different.

The common symptoms of high blood glucose are:

- Frequent urination
- Irritability
- Aggression
- Feeling very thirsty
- Dizziness/blurry vision
- Vomiting
- Unexplainable aches and pains

While the common symptoms of low blood glucose are:

- Shaking
- Blurry vision
- Racing heartbeat
- Feeling hungry, even if you're eating
- Feeling anxious/scared/defensive
- Fatigue
- Passing out

And a few general symptoms are:

- Cuts and bruises that take a long time to heal
- Headaches, especially from not eating
- Feeling thirsty often

Complications

When not properly managed, diabetes can lead to a number of serious complications. Uncontrolled diabetes (having frequent high blood glucose levels) can lead to nerve damage, known as neuropa-thy, meaning the hands, feet, and other body parts can experience numbness or tingling. Approximately 60–70% of patients report mild to severe cases of neuropathy. In severe cases, this may lead to amputation. More than 60% of nontrauma-related lower-limb amputations occurred because of this disease.

Other complications include erectile dysfunction, blindness (called retinopathy), heart disease, kidney disease, strokes, hearing loss, gum disease, mental health issues (anxiety and depression), and high blood pressure. In 2007, diabetes was listed as a relevant factor in 231,404 U.S. deaths.

Diagnosis

Diabetes is diagnosed one of three ways: the A1C Test; the fasting plasma glucose test; and the oral glucose tolerance test.

The A1C test, which assesses how much glucose has been in the blood over the past few months, is usually done through a blood drawing at a doctor's office. Nondiabetics test below 5.7, whereas above 6.5 indicates diabetes. Glucose levels in between these ranges considered "prediabetes," which means the body is becoming resis-tant to insulin.

In order to be tested using the fasting plasma glucose (FPG) test, the patient must fast and then has their blood glucose levels tested. Levels of less than 100 mg/dl are considered normal, while levels above 126 mg/dl are indicative of diabetes.

When a patient is administered the oral glucose tolerance test (OGTT), the patient eats a controlled amount of carbohydrates and then has his or her glucose tested after a brief period of time. Less than 140 mg/dl is normal while above 200 mg/dl indicates diabetes.

A glucometer or a home A1C test can be purchased at most phar-macies, though these are not necessarily accurate, and high num-bers on these do not mean someone definitely does or does not have diabetes. However, high readings on a home test can help convince a doctor that further testing needs to be done. Any concerns should be addressed with a professional, as they'll have access to the most reliable and accurate means of testing.

Risk Factors

As with any disease, there are a few major factors that can lead to developing diabetes. Genetics are a big component, and someone can be at much higher risk if a close family member has any meta-bolic disorder. This risk increases further if they have diabetes as well. Some minorities, most specifically African Americans and Latin Americans, tend to be at a higher risk as well.

A poor diet can contribute to developing diabetes specifically type 2 diabetes. If a person eats a foods that are high in calories and unhealthy fats, such as deserts and fast food, he or she risks gaining weight and increasing insulin resistance, as well as doing general damage to his or her body that may cause greater complications down the line, should that person develop diabetes. A diet high in fiber and vegetables can help to counter the risks of developing type 2 diabetes.

Additionally, a sedentary lifestyle can contribute to the develop-ment of diabetes. This is one of the reasons why it is important to get at least 30 minutes of exercise three days a week. Physical activ-ity not only helps to build muscle, strengthen the heart, and pro-mote good nutrient absorption, it helps to make sure one's body stays receptive to insulin.

Diseases affecting the pancreas, especially when young, as well as some types of infection, can lead to developing diabetes as well. People under age 40 are at greater risk for type 1 diabetes while those above age 45 are more likely to get type 2 diabetes. The older a woman is when she gets pregnant, the more likely she is to develop gestational diabetes. With an increasing number of women delay-ing motherhood in order to establish their careers, it is possible that the incidence of gestational diabetes may increase.

It's important to note that many prediabetics show heart and nerve damage as a result of poor glucose control, and this is before they officially have the disease. Accordingly, it is important to be healthy and active before symptoms arise.

Treatment

In prediabetics, treatment and, in some rare cases, reversal of warning signs can be achieved through increased exercise, good diet, and vitamin supplements. Avoiding alcohol can also help, as alcohol slows the metabolism and serves as empty, or unhealthy, calories. Junk food falls under the same "empty-calorie" category.

Type 1 diabetics control their blood glucose through use of a glucometer. Since their bodies don't produce insulin at all, they take shots or use an insulin pump to receive it throughout the day: short-acting insulin for food and long-acting insulin to keep their blood glucose from rising when not eating or active. Exercise is also effective for keeping glucose down.

Type 2 diabetics, in moderate cases, tend to control their disease and glucose levels through diet and exercise. In more advanced cases, they take insulin as well, though often orally as opposed to a shot.

Severe low or high blood glucose levels are often treated through hospitalization, where a staff can monitor the levels, stabilize them, and talk with the patient about why this happened and how to prevent it in the future.

DATA AND ANALYSES

Data

Table 22.1 Number (in thousands) of Civilian, Noninstitutionalized Persons With Diagnosed Diabetes, by Age: United States, 2001–2011

Year	Age group				
	0–44	45–64	65–74	75+	Total
2001	2233	5635	2931	2085	12884
2002	2213	6034	3054	2264	13566
2003	2217	6411	3201	2447	14275
2004	2417	6932	3331	2540	15221
2005	2733	7437	3428	2698	16295
2006	2823	7813	3577	2801	17014
2007	2801	8356	3750	2936	17842
2008	2893	9067	3962	3035	18958
2009	3100	9595	4204	3304	20202
2010	3149	9754	4510	3432	20845
2011	3017	9689	4712	3516	20934

Source: http://www.cdc.gov/diabetes/statistics/prev/national/tnumage.htm

Analysis

Table 22.1 demonstrates the increase of diabetes diagnosis by age range. The 0–44 age range, which is most likely to get type 1 diabetes, increased by roughly 800,000 diagnosed people in that period. However, the total number of diagnoses increased by eight million, leaving almost seven million diagnoses that are statistically more likely to have been type 2 diabetes. Since age alone cannot have caused such an increase, it is reasonable to conclude that people in these ranges are more susceptible to poor diet, stress, and a lack of exercise, indicating such adults may more information on how to prevent this disease.

Data

Table 22.2 Percentage of Civilian, Noninstitutionalized Persons With Diagnosed Diabetes, by Age, Race, and Sex: United States, 2011

| | | Age | | | | | | | |
| | | 0–44 | | 45–64 | | 65–74 | | 75+ | |
Race	Sex	%	Std error	%	Std error	Percent	Std error	%	Std error
White	M	1.5	0.11	12.4	0.47	22.8	1.04	21.7	1.02
	F	1.5	0.12	10.0	0.37	18.4	0.86	16.6	0.83
Black	M	2.5	0.30	17.6	1.25	30.7	2.33	38.1	3.47
	F	2.4	0.29	17.1	0.98	31.2	2.39	25.9	1.80
Asian	M	1.4	0.38	12.7	1.92	34.4	4.28	30.4	5.91
	F	1.0	0.29	11.3	1.66	18.3	3.40	18.7	4.08

Source: http://www.cdc.gov/diabetes/statistics/prev/national/fig2004.htm

Analysis

As seen in Table 22.2, Black people are significantly more likely to be diagnosed with diabetes, especially in the 65–74 and 75+ age ranges, though age 45–64 is high as well. Asian women do not tend to be significantly different from white women and are diagnosed less than black women, though Asian men face higher diagnosis rates than white men. This points to a genetic predisposition among black people to develop diabetes—one that Asian men older than 64 may suffer from as well.

Data

Table 22.3 Number of Emergency Room Visits Due to Diabetes, All Ages, 2006–2009

Year	Number (in thousands)
2006	9,464
2007	10,149
2008	10,907
2009	11,492

Source: http://www.cdc.gov/diabetes/statistics/emergency/fig1.htm

Analysis

Table 22.3 shows that two million more people were admitted to the hospital due to diabetes-related concerns in 2006 than 2009. This is placing a huge toll on our medical system. In fact, recent data shows that diabetes is responsible for $116 billion in direct medical costs annually.[1] This data demonstrates that more education on diabetes is necessary, as people are unable to recognize the symptoms of this disease earlier on and effectively manage their disease prior to the development of more severe symptoms that may require hospitalization.

DISCUSSION QUESTIONS

1. Table 22.1 shows that diabetes diagnoses are increasing over the years and, generally, across age levels, what are some possible reasons for this?
2. The data presented in Table 22.2 show that African Americans are more likely than Asians or whites to develop diabetes. Given this data, do you think our health system should offer diabetes detection and prevention strategies that are more targeted toward the African American community? If so, what are some strategies that can be used?
3. A considerable number of pregnant women develop gestational diabetes, what additional measures should obstetricians take to ensure that their patients are taking adequate measures to prevent the development of diabetes?
4. Table 22.3 shows that two million more people were admitted to the hospital due to diabetes related concerns in 2006 than 2009. What can our public health system due to reduce the number of diabetes-related hospitalizations?
5. A number of lifestyle factors, including diet and physical activity levels may contribute to the development of type 2 diabetes. What can be done to motivate individuals to adopt healthier lifestyles in order to reduce the risk of type 2 diabetes?

---

[1] Geri Aston, "Diabetes, an Alarming Epidemic," *Hospitals & Health Networks*, Feb 1, 2013, http://www.hhnmag.com/display/HHN-news-article.dhtml?dcrPath=/templatedata/HF_Common/NewsArticle/data/HHN/Magazine/2013/Feb/0213HHN_Feature_chroniccare.

23

DIGESTIVE DISEASES

INTRODUCTION

Understanding Digestive Diseases

Digestion occurs when the body breaks down food in order to create and nourish cells that provide energy. Digestive diseases affect digestion and the digestive tract, also known as the gastrointestinal tract. The digestive system is made up of various organs joined in a long, twisted tube, starting with the mouth. Next is the esophagus, stomach, small and large intestines, and finally, the anus. The liver, gallbladder, and pancreas are also part of the digestive system, as they secrete fluids to aid digestion.

Digestive diseases can range from common conditions such as acid reflux, to life-threatening diseases such as cancer. Common digestive disorders are categorized by which organ they affect:

- Rectal disorders include anal fissures, hemorrhoids, and proctitis
- Esophageal disorders include narrowing and achalasia
- Liver disorders include hepatitis B and C, cirrhosis, and liver failure
- Pancreatic disorders include pancreatitis

- Intestinal disorders include celiac disease, Crohn's disease, ulcerative colitis, diverticulitis, and short bowel syndrome
- Additional disorders include irritable bowel syndrome, lactose intolerance, gastroesophageal reflux disease, and hiatal hernia

Symptoms

Symptoms vary depending on the type and severity of digestive diseases; however, common symptoms include:

- Blood in stool
- Changes in bowel habits
- Bloating
- Diarrhea
- Constipation
- Severe abdominal pain, nausea, or vomiting
- Unintentional weight gain or loss
- Heartburn
- Difficulty swallowing

It is important to contact a medical professional if any gastrointestinal symptoms are experienced, as the cause of the symptoms can range from common conditions to life-threatening diseases.

Risk Factors

Many conditions are categorized as digestive diseases; therefore, the causes and risk factors often vary. Consistent factors that increase the risk of developing digestive diseases include:

- Eating foods that irritate the digestive system, including high-fat diets
- Stress
- Radiation therapy
- Alcohol abuse
- Abdominal trauma
- Medications, especially overuse of aspirin
- Obesity
- Pregnancy
- Smoking

Additionally, certain gastrointestinal problems can lead to additional digestive diseases. Conditions such as Crohn's disease, ulcerative colitis, and gastrointestinal cancers often increase the risk of developing other digestive diseases.

Diagnosis

Physical examinations and medical history help health care professionals diagnose digestive disorders. Some disorders require extensive evaluations before diagnosis, involving laboratory tests, imaging tests, or endoscopic procedures.

Laboratory tests that may be used to diagnose digestive diseases include fecal occult blood tests, which check for hidden blood in the stool, and stool cultures, which check for the presence of abnormal bacteria in the digestive tract.

Imaging tests may be used to examine how food moves throughout the body, such as ingesting barium so a radiologist can view the stomach's digestion of the meal; colorectal transit studies that observes food as it passes through the colon; or ingesting a radioisotope that shows food passing through the stomach. Other imaging tests include computed tomography scans (CT scan), ultrasounds, and magnetic resonance imaging (MRI) that examine various parts of the body; defecographies, which examine the anorectal area with an X-ray; lower gastrointestinal (GI) series or barium enemas, which examine the rectum, large intestine, and part of the small intestine with an X-ray; and upper GI series or barium swallows, which examine the esophagus, stomach, and duodenum.

Endoscopic procedures include colonoscopies, endoscopic retrograde cholangiopancreatographies (ERCP), esophagogastroduodenoscopies (EGD), and sigmoidoscopies. Colonoscopies use a colonoscope that is inserted into the rectum to examine the large intestine and identify abnormalities such as inflammation, ulcers, or bleeding. ERCPs use X-rays to guide an endoscope through the mouth and down to the esophagus, stomach, and duodenum. ERCPs are typically done when patients present problems with the liver, gallbladder, bile ducts, and pancreas. An EGD is a similar process, using an endoscope to examine the esophagus, stomach, and duodenum. Sigmoidoscopies insert a sigmoidoscope into the rectum to inflate and examine the large intestine for abnormalities.

Additional tests that may be used for diagnosis include anorectal manometries, esophageal manometries, and gastric manometries that measure the strength of the muscles in different parts of the digestive system. Overall, the types of diagnostic procedures will depend on the type and severity of the digestive disease.

Treatment

Some digestive diseases can be treated with a change in diet or prescription medications; however, other conditions may require greater measures. In addition to avoiding high-fat, acidic foods, other lifestyle changes that may help relieve symptoms include quitting smoking, limiting alcohol consumption, and exercising regularly. Over-the-counter medications such as antacids and pain relievers can treat less severe digestive diseases, as well as prescription medications and antibiotics.

More serious digestive diseases may require hospitalization, where IV fluids, stomach draining, and further assessments can be completed. Surgery is common when treating the digestive tract. Procedures can be done various ways, including endoscopic, laparoscopic, and open surgery. Organs transplants of the liver, pancreas, and small intestine are also common. Radiation or chemotherapy may also be used to treat severe digestive diseases, such as gastrointestinal cancers.

DATA AND ANALYSES

Data

Table 23.1 Deaths, Ambulatory Care Visits, and Hospital Discharges of Digestive Diseases: United States, 2004

Digestive disease	Deaths	Ambulatory care visits	Hospital discharges
All digestive diseases	236,164	104,790,000	13,533,000
All digestive cancer	135,107	4,198,000	726,000
Liver disease	36,090	2,398,000	759,000
All viral hepatitis	5,393	3,510,000	475,000
Gastrointestinal infections	4,396	2,365,000	450,000
Peptic ulcer disease	3,692	1,473,000	489,000
Pancreatitis	3,480	881,000	454,000
Diverticular disease	3,372	3,269,000	815,000
Abdominal wall hernia	1,172	4,787,000	372,000
Gastroesophageal reflux disease	1,150	18,342,000	3,189,000

Source: Everhart, J.E. 2008. "Burden of digestive diseases in the United States report." National Institutes of Health. Retrieved from: http://www.niddk.nih.gov/about-niddk/strategic-plans-reports/Pages/burden-digestive-diseases-in-united-states-report.aspx#Index

Analysis

Table 23.1 presents deaths, ambulatory care visits, and hospital discharges related to digestive diseases. Liver disease and four types of gastrointestinal cancers each caused over 10,000 deaths. Transmissible infectious diseases, including gastrointestinal infections and hepatitis accounted for the a significant number of deaths as well.

The digestive diseases most responsible for ambulatory care visits included gastroesophageal reflux disease (GERD), abdominal wall hernia, gastrointestinal cancers, hepatitis, and diverticular disease. The digestive diseases most responsible for hospital visits included GERD, diverticular disease, liver disease, and gastrointestinal cancers.

Overall, the data stated that over 230,000 individuals in the United States die each year because of digestive diseases, in addition to over 100 million individuals requiring ambulatory care visits and 13.5 million individuals requiring hospital stays. Further research can examine the leading causes of deaths, ambulatory visits, and hospitalizations related to digestive diseases.

Data

Table 23.2 Prevalence of Gastrointestinal Symptoms Across Body Mass Index (BMI) Categories for Each Symptom of Gastroesophageal Reflux Disease (GERD): United States, 2008

BMI category	BMI	Percentage with nausea	Percentage with vomiting	Percentage with regurgitation	Percentage with heart burn
Underweight	<18.5	7.1	0.0	—	—
Normal weight	18.5–24.9	7.9	1.2	4.4	11.4
Overweight	25–25.9	6.8	1.5	7.8	14.2
Obese class I	30–34.9	10.6	3.0	5.2	25.3
Obese class II	35–39.9	10.7	7.1	5.6	16.0
Obese class III	>40	10.0	6.7	20.0	25.0

Source: Chaudry, N.U., Haque, I.U., Rehman, A.U., Tayyab, G.U.N., & Zafar, S. 2008. "Correlation of gastroesophageal reflux disease symptoms with body mass index." Retrieved from: http://www.ncbi.nlm.nih.gov/pmc/articles/PMC2702902/

Analysis

Gastroesophageal reflux disease (GERD) accounts for a significant amount of ambulatory care visits and hospitalizations each year, as it is a common digestive disease; however, GERD is not a severe condition and can be treated with changes in diet. Table 23.2 presents the prevalence of gastrointestinal symptoms related to GERD across body mass index (BMI) categories. Using the World Health Organization guidelines to determine body weight classifications, BMI is a calculation of the relative body weight for height. The data presented that the majority of symptoms related to GERD increase directly with BMI. Heartburn was the most common symptom, followed by regurgitation. The finding presents the importance of nutritional education and decreasing obesity rates in the United States. By decreasing the amount of overweight and obese individuals, the ambulatory care visit and hospitalization rates related to GERD should also decrease.

Data

Table 23.3 Deaths, Ambulatory Care Visits, and Hospital Discharges of Digestive Cancers: United States, 2004

Digestive disease	Deaths	Ambulatory care visits	Hospital discharges
All digestive diseases	236,164	104,790,000	13,533,000
All digestive cancer	135,107	4,198,000	726,000
Colorectal cancer	53,226	2,589,000	255,000
Pancreatic cancer	31,800	415,000	68,000
Esophageal cancer	13,667	372,000	44,000
Gastric cancer	11,253	141,000	31,000
Primary liver cancer	6,323	63,000	33,000
Bile duct cancer	4,954	—	17,000
Gallbladder cancer	1,939	—	9,000
Cancer of the small intestine	1,115	—	9,000

Source: Chaudry, N.U., Haque, I.U., Rehman, A.U., Tayyab, G.U.N., & Zafar, S. 2008. "Correlation of gastroesophageal reflux disease symptoms with body mass index." Retrieved from: http://www.ncbi.nlm.nih.gov/pmc/articles/PMC2702902/

Analysis

Table 23.3 further examines the deaths, ambulatory care visits, and hospital discharges related to digestive diseases by focusing specifically on the leading cause of death, digestive cancers. By examining the most common gastrointestinal cancers, the data presented that colorectal cancer and pancreatic cancer account for more than two times the amount of deaths than other digestive cancers.

Similarly, these two types of digestive cancer related to the highest ambulatory care visits and hospitalizations. Less severe digestive cancers included esophageal cancer, gastric cancer, and primary liver cancer.

Data

Table 23.4 Percentage of Colorectal Cancer Diagnoses Over a Ten-interval by Current Age and Gender: United States, 2008–2010

Current age	Percentage of male diagnoses	Percentage of female diagnoses
30	0.07	0.07
40	0.25	0.22
50	0.69	0.53
60	1.32	0.92
70	2.08	1.61

Source: Division of Cancer Prevention and Control. 2013. "Colorectal (colon) cancer." Centers for Disease Control and Prevention. Retrieved from: http://www.cdc.gov/cancer/colorectal/statistics/age.htm

Analysis

Colorectal cancer accounts for the most deaths, ambulatory care visits, and hospitalizations of all digestive cancers. Table 23.4 examines the percentage of diagnoses over a ten-year interval by current age and gender. For example, it is estimated that 1.32% of 60-year-old males will be diagnosed with colorectal cancer by the age of 70. This percentage amounts to 1 or 2 out of every 100 males who are currently 60 years old. From examining the rates, it is apparent that the risk of developing colorectal cancer increases with age and is slightly greater in males than females. Further examination can compare these rates with other digestive cancers to determine overall risk factors and estimate future prevalence.

DISCUSSION QUESTIONS

1. How can the number of ambulatory care visits related to digestive diseases be decreased? Would education about gastrointestinal symptoms and the importance of seeking a medical diagnosis help prevent the number of ambulatory care visits in the United States?

2. Why does gastroesophageal reflux disease (GERD) present such high ambulatory care visits and hospitalizations, even though it is not one of the most severe digestive diseases? What treatment methods can be used for GERD to lower these numbers?

3. How can liver disease and gastrointestinal cancers be detected sooner? Will early diagnosis help decrease the mortality rate related to these digestive diseases?

4. Why do colorectal and pancreatic cancer account for over two times the amount of deaths than other gastrointestinal cancers? How can these mortality rates be reduced?

5. Why do colorectal cancer rates increase with age? Additionally, why are more males diagnosed with colorectal cancer than females? How do these rates compare to other?

24

DISABILITIES

INTRODUCTION

Understanding Disabilities

A disability is a broad term that refers to any mental or physical health condition that limits a person's capacity to perform certain functions. There are many types of disabilities, each of which has the potential to obstruct what is considered normal, comfortable execution of everyday tasks. Disabilities can affect a person's ability to:

- Hear
- See
- Move
- Think
- Remember
- Learn
- Communicate
- Maintain mental health
- Engage fully in social relationships

Disabilities in general differ from other diseases, conditions, and illnesses because everything from diagnosis, causes, and risk factors, among other aspects, is not clear-cut and usually depends on the unique situation of the individual with the disability.

Causes

There are many different kinds of disabilities that affect different areas of the body or mind. It is no surprise then that there are countless different factors that cause them. Some of these have the potential to produce more than one disability at a time.

It is important to note that any person can either be born with a disability, or develop one after they are born as a result of uncontrollable factors like age, genetics, or an accident. For example, a person who cannot see might have been born with an ocular condition, or they might have been able to see before suffering a vision-impairing accident as a child or adult. Likewise, a person might not have full mobility of their legs if they were born with a debilitating disease, or if they developed the same or a similar disease later in life, resulting in paralysis or amputation of those legs.

Treatment

Because a person's age, health, and stage of disability is unique to them, it goes without saying that any way of coping with or treating their disability will be different from anyone else's. Therefore, it is crucial for a person with a disability to consult a doctor, specialist, or other health care provider for personalized treatment that will work for him or her. Treatment for a disability, depending on the type, can come in the form of surgery, medication, physical therapy, and support groups, among many others.

Sometimes, treatment cannot fully "cure" a disability, but it can make living with a disability more comfortable or bearable for a person. With advances in technology, many devices have become available for people with intellectual and developmental disabilities to aid them with living at home and in a community, working, learning, being healthy and safe, and engaging in social activities. Just some of the most common assistive technologies used for these purposes include:

- Speech-generating devices
- Screen magnifiers
- Audiobooks
- Beeping crosswalk signals
- Refreshable braille displays
- Video job training
- Wheelchair-accessible public transportation
- Exercise videos

- Picture-based books and e-mails
- Closed captioning
- Augmentative communication devices
- Alert or alarm watches and phones
- Emergency alarms that can be seen and heard
- Online programs

Whether or not treatment can be administered to fully reverse a disability, doctors usually stress the importance of physical activity. Of course, the amount of physical activity a person with a disability engages in depends on their abilities and fitness level—specifically, how long or strenuously they can exercise without becoming overwhelmed.

The Centers for Disease Control and Prevention suggests several physical activities for people with disabilities to participate in. These activities include but are not limited to:

- Wheeling oneself in a wheelchair
- Wheelchair basketball, tennis, football, or softball
- Aquatic therapy
- Brisk walking
- Hand-crank bicycling
- Hiking
- Horseback riding
- Nordic walking
- Rowing
- Seated volleyball
- Swimming laps
- Water aerobics

DATA AND ANALYSES

Data

Table 24.1 Percentage of People in the United States of All Ages With Disability Status by State, 2004

Percentage of people with disabilities	States
1–10.9	U.S. Virgin Islands
11–15.9	California, District of Columbia, Iowa, North Dakota

(Continued)

Table 24.1 Percentage of People in the United States of All Ages With Disability Status by State, 2004 (*Continued*)

Percentage of people with disabilities	States
16–20.9	Alabama, Alaska, Arizona, Arkansas, Colorado, Connecticut, Delaware, Florida, Georgia, Idaho, Illinois, Indiana, Kansas, Louisiana, Maine, Maryland, Massachusetts, Montana, Nebraska, Nevada, New Hampshire, New Jersey, New Mexico, New York, North Carolina, Ohio, Pennsylvania, Rhode Island, South Carolina, South Dakota, Tennessee, Texas, Utah, Vermont, Virginia, Wisconsin, Wyoming
≥21	Kentucky, Michigan, Minnesota, Mississippi, Missouri, Oklahoma, Oregon, Puerto Rico, Washington, West Virginia
Data not available	Guam, Hawaii

Source: http://dhds.cdc.gov/dataviews/tabular?viewId=792&geoId=1&subsetId=&z=1

Analysis

Table 24.1 shows the percentage of people in the United States with disability status by state in 2004. The states with recorded data fell into the 1–10.9%, 11–15.9%, 16–20.9%, or ≥21% ranges.

In 2004, 32 of the 52 states with recorded data (more than two-thirds of the total) featured a percentage of people with disabilities between 16% and 20.9%.

Data

Table 24.2 Percentage of People in the United States of All Ages With Disability Status by state, 2011

Percentage of people with disabilities	States
1–10.9	none
11–15.9	none
16–20.9	Hawaii, Iowa, Minnesota, New Jersey, Puerto Rico
≥21	Alabama, Alaska, Arizona, Arkansas, California, Colorado, Connecticut, Delaware, District of Columbia, Florida, Georgia, Idaho, Illinois, Indiana, Kansas, Kentucky, Louisiana, Maine, Maryland, Massachusetts, Michigan, Mississippi, Missouri, Montana, Nebraska, Nevada, New Hampshire, New Mexico, New York, North Carolina,

Percentage of people with disabilities	States
Data not available	North Dakota, Ohio, Oklahoma, Oregon, Pennsylvania, Rhode Island, South Carolina, South Dakota, Tennessee, Texas, Utah, Vermont, Virginia, Washington, West Virginia, Wisconsin, Wyoming Guam, U.S. Virgin Islands

Source: http://dhds.cdc.gov/dataviews/tabular?viewId=792&geoId=1&subsetId=&z=1

Analysis

Table 24.2 expands on the data in the previous 2004 table, showing the percentage of people in the United States with disability status by state seven years later in 2011. The data shows a massive increase in the percentage of people with disabilities. In fact, every state's percentages increased significantly from 2004. Additionally, none of the states fell into the first two percentage ranges of 1–10.9% and 11–15.9%.

In 2011, 47 of the 52 states with recorded data (more than three-quarters of the total) featured a percentage of people with disabilities greater than 21%. The remaining five states all fell into the 16–20.9% range.

DISCUSSION QUESTIONS

1. There are several types of disabilities, each of which comes with its own difficulties and obstacles. Pick a disability related to the first list above. What challenges might a person with this disability encounter on a daily basis?
2. Despite the myriad of treatment options and assistive technologies available, a lack of disability-friendly environments can make living normally difficult for people with disabilities. What can stores, restaurants, offices, beaches, and similar locations do to allow people with disabilities to access, use, and navigate these places easily, safely, and comfortably?
3. Doctors usually recommend that people with all types of disabilities remain physically active. In fact, a popular phrase among doctors is "exercise is medicine." Why is being physically active important for people with disabilities?

4. The data in the tables above show a significant increase in percentage of people with disabilities in the United States from 2004 to 2011. What factors might account for this change in an overwhelming majority of states?

5. Surgery is just one of the many treatment options for people with disabilities. What disability can you think of that surgery would be key in reversing?

25

DRUG ADDICTION

INTRODUCTION

Understanding Drug Addiction

Drug addiction is defined as the compulsive use of drugs, despite knowing or consciously experiencing the harmful consequences of those drugs. Although many people do not acknowledge drug addiction as a health problem, it is actually considered a serious brain disease. This is because becoming addicted to drugs makes significant alterations to the structure and functioning of the brain over time. In fact, scientists have found that drug addiction decreases brain metabolism and affects the parts of the brain that deal with making decisions. The latter explains why it becomes increasingly difficult for a person to exercise self-control on what started as a voluntary action.

Drug addiction extends to any type of drug, whether a person is taking them for medical reasons, to feel good, or to do a task better. Some of these drugs include:

- Nicotine
- Alcohol
- Marijuana
- Inhalants
- Cocaine
- Amphetamines

- Ecstasy
- LSD
- Heroin
- Steroids
- Prescription Medications

Signs and Symptoms

Throughout the course of a drug addiction, a person can experience physical and mental changes that are either short-term or long-term and can extend to home, school, and the workplace. These signs and symptoms can usually help signal to family members, friends, or community leaders that the person is suffering from drug addiction and should seek help. Just some of the signs and symptoms of drug addiction include:

- Strongly feeling the need to use the drug often
- Using the drug to cope with problems
- Maintaining a constant supply of the drug
- Failing to stop use of the drug
- Deterioration of close friendships or relationships
- Deterioration of hygiene
- Mood swings
- Apathy
- Anxiety
- Sudden weight loss or gain
- Bloodshot eyes or dilated pupils
- Chronically inflamed nostrils

Although some of these signs and symptoms of drug addiction may seem similar to those of other diseases, illnesses, or conditions, a combination of them is usually a clear indicator of a drug problem.

Diagnosis

Diagnosis of a drug addiction does not involve the use of blood tests or biopsies. Instead, a doctor, psychiatrist, psychologist, and/ or an addiction counselor evaluate a patient on their frequency of drug use and behavior. One or more of these medical professionals must make certain that the individual meets the criteria listed in the *Diagnostic and Statistical Manual of Mental Disorders* (5th ed.; American Psychiatric Association, 2013). The criteria in this manual include but are not limited to the build-up of tolerance to a drug over time, appearance of withdrawal symptoms, taking increasingly larger amounts of a drug, and replacing important events or activities to take a drug.

Risk Factors

Although drug addiction can impact anyone, regardless of their age, gender, race, or ethnicity, there are certain risk factors that make some individuals especially vulnerable to it. While not a single one of these factors, whether they are brought on by the individual, their friends, family, or community, guarantees drug addiction, they all put others more at risk for the brain changes associated with addiction. The risk factors that are connected to drug addiction include:

- Early use
- Poverty
- Poor social skills
- Lack of parental supervision
- Curiosity
- Peer pressure
- Substance abuse
- Drug availability

Luckily, drug addiction is a preventable health problem. With each risk factor comes a protective factor that can counter the threat of potential drug addiction. Some examples of protective factors for drug addiction include anti-drug policies, educational programs that clearly outline the negative effects of drugs, and parental supervision and support.

Effects

It goes without saying that a drug addiction can have disastrous effects on the people an addicted person comes into contact with, whether that is secondhand smoke or death or injury from drugged driving. The most disastrous consequences, however, are usually brought on to the individual themselves. People addicted to drugs usually find themselves more susceptible to life-altering medical events, including:

- Cardiovascular disease
- Depression
- Cancer

- HIV/AIDS
- Lung disease
- Brain damage
- Stroke
- Hepatitis B and C
- Mental disorders
- Death as a result of these events

Treatment

Drug addiction is not just a preventable health problem; it is also a treatable one, once it is diagnosed and assessed. Unfortunately, treatment is not as simple as going through a weeklong or month-long medical detoxification that cleans the drug out of the patient's body and guides the patient through withdrawal. This is mainly due to the fact that there are so many different drugs and each individual is at a different stage in their addiction to one or more of those drugs. However, treatment usually entails a combination of medication and behavioral therapy for an extended period of time.

In the United States, there are several pills, patches, and lozenges, as well as prescription versions of these medications, approved by the Food and Drug Administration to treat opioid, tobacco, and alcohol addictions. However, it can be very risky—even counterproductive—to treat drug addiction with medication. The individual has the potential to become addicted to what is meant to work against their existing drug addiction.

Behavioral therapy can help in this regard, as it can help the individual acknowledge the negative effects of drug addiction and instill a sense of positivity and readiness to make a lifestyle change.

DATA AND ANALYSES

Data

Table 25.1 Number of Americans Aged 12 or Older Who Used an Illicit Drug or Psychotherapeutic Medication in the Past Month, 2012

Drug	Number
Marijuana	18,900,000
Psychotherapeutic	6,800,000
Cocaine	1,600,000
Hallucinogens	1,100,000

Drug	Number
Inhalants	500,000
Heroin	300,000

Source: National Institute of Drug Abuse, DrugFacts: Nationwide Trends. Retrieved from: http://www.drugabuse.gov/publications/drugfacts/nationwide-trends

Analysis

Table 25.1 outlines the number of Americans aged 12 or older who abused illicit drugs or psychotherapeutic medication in the month before the survey was taken. Marijuana revealed the highest number, with 18.9 million abusers. This is almost triple that of the 6.8 million psychotherapeutic medication abusers. The data runs alongside the fact that marijuana use in the United States has been steadily increasing over the years, much more than other illicit drugs like those in the table.

Data

Table 25.2 Specific Illicit Drug Dependence or Abuse in the Past Year Among Persons Aged 12 or Older, 2012

Drug	Number
Marijuana	4,304,000
Pain relievers	2,056,000
Cocaine	1,119,000
Tranquilizers	629,000
Stimulants	535,000
Heroin	467,000
Hallucinogens	331,000
Inhalants	164,000
Sedatives	135,000

Source: Substance Abuse and Mental Health Administration, Results from the 2012 National Survey on Drug Use and Health (NSDUH). Retrieved from: http://www.samhsa.gov/data/NSDUH/2012SummNatFindDetTables/NationalFindings/NSDUHresults2012.htm

Analysis

Table 25.2 shows the dependence and abuse of certain drugs by Americans in the year before the survey was taken. Marijuana is well ahead of all other illicit drugs, with 4.3 million dependent users or abusers—more than double that of about 2.1 million pain reliever dependent users and abusers. This is an important supplement to Table 25.1, as it shows the prevalence of marijuana and its increase in use correlates with an increase in its abuse.

Data

Table 25.3 Percentage of Admissions to Publicly Funded Substance Abuse Treatment Programs by Age, 2008

Age group	Percentage
25–29 years	14.8%
20–24 years	14.4%
40–44 years	12.6%
35–39 years	11.7%
45–49 years	11.5%
30–34 years	11.3%
50–59 years	10.4%
12–17 years	7.5%
18–19 years	4.1%
60–64 years	1.2%
≥65 years	0.6%

Source: http://www.drugabuse.gov/publications/drugfacts/treatment-statistics

Analysis

Table 25.3 shows the percentage of Americans admitted to abuse treatment programs in 2008. The data, which primarily takes into account the age of admitted patients, is arranged starting with the highest percentage age group and decreasing for each consecutive age group.

In general, there was no consistent trend between the age groups. Individuals aged between 25 to 29 years who were addicted to one or more drugs showed the highest percentage of admission, 14.8%. Those aged 65 or older, on the other hand, showed the lowest percentage of admission, 0.6%.

DISCUSSION QUESTIONS

1. Some people are less susceptible to drug addiction than others. What aspects of health or history would possibly explain

why a teenage white girl is less prone to addiction than an addicted teenage white girl in the same town?

2. Although many people think of drugs such as cocaine or heroin when it comes to drug addiction, the condition also extends to alcohol. Why is alcohol considered a drug?

3. Early use, poverty, and lack of parental supervision are three of the many risk factors associated with drug addiction. Using a real-world scenario, how might these risk factors work together to develop into a drug addiction?

4. There is a countless number of signs and symptoms of drug addiction, whether they are short term, long term, physical, mental, or behavioral. Aside from those listed above, what are some other signs and symptoms of drug addiction, and what drug in particular might they be associated with?

5. Marijuana has the highest rate of dependence or abuse among all other drugs. What are some possible reasons for this?

26

EATING DISORDERS

INTRODUCTION

Understanding Eating Disorders

Eating disorders are a group of illnesses focused on the consumption of food. Eating disorders are distinguished by persistent disturbances in eating or eating-related behavior that result in the altered consumption or absorption of food. Eating disorders can significantly impair physical health and social functioning. If left untreated, eating disorders have the potential to result in death.

The Diagnostic and Statistical Manual of Mental Disorders (5th ed.; American Psychiatric Association, 2013) has expanded the category of eating disorders. Currently, there are nine categories of identifiable and diagnosable eating disorders. The most common eating disorders are anorexia nervosa, bulimia nervosa, and binge-eating disorder. Less common eating disorders are avoidant/restrictive food intake disorder, rumination disorder, pica, other specified feeding or eating disorders, and unspecified feeding or eating disorders. Other specified eating disorders are categorized by behaviors that do not meet the full criteria of one of the recognized, diagnosable eating disorders.

Anorexia nervosa and bulimia nervosa involve extreme fear of weight gain, coupled with behaviors designed to alter food consumption and absorption. Anorexia nervosa is categorized by an inadequate food intake that results in a low weight; however, atypical anorexia nervosa is also recognized as a specified eating disorder, in which an individual's weight is not below normal even though the individual poses symptoms of anorexia nervosa. Bulimia nervosa is categorized by frequent episodes of binging, followed by extreme measures to prevent weight gain, such as self-induced vomiting. Other specified eating disorders related to bulimia nervosa include bulimia nervosa with less frequent behaviors and purging disorder, in which an individual self-induces vomiting without binging beforehand.

Binge-eating disorder is distinguished by recurrent and regular (on average once a week) episodes of binge eating without the follow-up of measures to prevent weight gain. Binge-eating is defined by consuming an excessive amount of food that is disproportionately larger than what most people would eat in a similar time period under similar circumstances. Other specified eating disorders related to binge-eating disorder include binge-eating disorder of lesser frequency and night eating syndrome, in which an individual excessively consumes food at nighttime.

Avoidant/restrictive food intake disorder is characterized by an apparent avoidance or restriction of food intake, which results in a failure to meet nutritional needs. Rumination disorder is marked by the repeated regurgitation of food, while pica is characterized by the eating of one or more nonnutritive, nonfood substances. Unspecified eating disorders are categorized by behaviors that do not meet the criteria of other feeding and eating disorders, but still cause serious clinical damage. Additionally, unspecified eating disorders can be diagnosed when a medical professional does not have enough information about an individual's eating behaviors, such as in an emergency situation.

Symptoms

Anorexia Nervosa

- Restriction of food intake relative to nutritional requirements, leading to a significantly low body weight
- Intense fear of weight gain or "becoming fat", recurrent behavior that interferes and inhibits weight gain and preoccupation with weight, food, and calories
- Development of food rituals and excuses to hide the lack of consumption

- Disturbance and distortion in the perception of one's body weight or shape
- Excessive exercise regardless of fatigue, illness, or injury
- Withdrawal from friends, family, and normal activities
- Heightened influence of body weight or shape on self-evaluation
- Refusal to acknowledge the severity of significantly low body weight

Bulimia Nervosa

- Recurrent episodes of binge-eating
- Sense of a lack of control during binge eating episodes
- Recurrent and compensatory behaviors performed to prevent weight gain (e.g., vomiting, use of laxatives, diuretics, fasting, excessive exercise) following binge-eating episodes
- Heightened influence of body shape and weight on self-evaluation
- Withdrawal from friends, family, and normal activities
- Unusual swelling of the cheeks and jaw
- Calluses on the back of hands and knuckles from self-induced vomiting
- Discoloration or staining of teeth from self-induced vomiting

Binge-Eating Disorder

- Recurrent episodes of binge-eating that are not followed by behaviors designed to prevent weight gain
- Feeling a sense of lack of control during binge-eating episodes
- Feelings of shame or guilt typically follow an episode

Avoidant/Restrictive Food Intake Disorder

- Avoidance or restriction of food intake
- Inability to meet nutritional or energy needs
- Food related behaviors are not accompanied by psychological symptoms seen in anorexia nervosa

Rumination Disorder

- Repeated regurgitation of food that has already been swallowed
- Regurgitated food may be spit out, rechewed, or reswallowed

Pica

- Recurrent eating of nonnutritive, nonfood substances
- Behavior is not considered culturally or socially accepted
- May occur with another mental disorder (e.g., intellectual disability, autism spectrum disorder, schizophrenia)

Eating disorders can pose serious medical complications, and become life threatening if left untreated. Aside from malnutrition and significantly low body weight, anorexia nervosa can lead to a slow heart rate, low blood pressure, amenorrhea, muscle loss and weakness, decrease in bone density (brittle bones), severe dehydration, dry hair and skin, hair loss, starvation, and even cardiac arrest. Bulimia nervosa can induce an electrolyte imbalance, gastrointestinal problems (e.g., gastric ulcers), gastric ruptures, esophageal tears, cardiac arrhythmias, menstrual irregularity or amenorrhea, and tooth staining and decay. Potential health problems that can arise from binge-eating disorder include: high blood pressure, high cholesterol levels, heart disease, diabetes mellitus, gallbladder disease, and musculoskeletal problems.

Diagnosis

A variety of professionals can diagnose eating disorders. Mental health professionals (psychiatrists, psychologists, mental health counselors, and social workers) typically diagnose eating disorders, however a family doctor or pediatrician may make a diagnosis after observing symptoms. Individuals with eating disorders rarely seek out medical care on their own, so concerned parents, family, or friends typically schedule an assessment for the individual. There are no laboratory or blood tests to specifically screen for an eating disorder. If an eating disorder has manifested to produce additional medical symptoms and complications, medical professionals can use a variety of medical tests to gauge the severity (e.g., blood work, bone-density exam, electrocardiogram). When considering a diagnosis of anorexia nervosa, clinicians will focus on the individual's body mass index (BMI), which is a measure of body weight and height derived from the World Health Organization derived to outline healthy body weight according to height. BMI categories range from obese to underweight. Professionals can use a variety of assessment tools and questionnaires when interviewing an individual with a possible eating disorder. Questions will typically focus on current eating habits, body weight, recent weight loss or gain, as well as personal views on weight and body image. Questions may be supplemented with a focus on physical symptoms that may be associated with an eating disorder (e.g., constantly feeling cold, bruising easily, fatigue, or fainting).

The current diagnostic criteria for eating disorders can be found in the *Diagnostic and Statistical Manual of Mental Disorders* (5th ed.; American Psychiatric Association, 2013). Although psychiatrists and other mental health professionals developed this criteria, medical clinicians also use it. Each individual eating disorder is provided with specific diagnostic criteria. In order to reach an eating disorder diagnosis, the food related behaviors and eating disturbances cannot be attributed to a medical condition (e.g., gastrointestinal diseases, esophageal reflux, acquired immunodeficiency syndrome [AIDS]). Additionally, the food-related behaviors cannot be explained or substantiated by social or cultural practice.

Risk Factors

Eating disorders affect individuals from a variety of backgrounds and are acknowledged to be a serious, potentially life threatening illness. Eating disorders accumulate from a combination of psychological, interpersonal, social, and biological, factors. Some potential risk factors have been identified.

- Psychological factors: Depression, anxiety, stress, low self-esteem, loneliness, feelings of inadequacy
- Interpersonal factors: History of being ridiculed over weight, history of physical or sexual abuse, difficulty expressing emotions, troubled personal relationships
- Social factors: Cultural pressures that glorify "thinness," cultural norms that value people based on physical appearance, stress related to discrimination based on physical characteristics such as race or weight
- Biological: Gender—females tend to be at a higher risk than males; current research is studying chemical imbalances and genetics related to the development of eating disorders

Treatment

Eating disorders require psychological treatment conjoined with appropriate medical care in order to foster recovery. Medical care is crucial to ensure the individual is meeting basic nutritional needs, while psychological counseling is needed to assist individuals in addressing the symptoms contributing to the eating disorder. Underlying psychological, interpersonal, and cultural forces may play a role in the manifestation of an eating disorder. Eating disorders are complex illnesses that vary on a case-by-case basis and best respond to an individualized treatment plan.

Mental health professionals typically provide treatment and care for eating disorders, however treatment may also involve medical doctors and nutritionists. Individuals with eating disorders typically respond to outpatient therapy such as individual, group, or family therapy, support groups, nutritional counseling, and psychiatric medications when needed. Medication coupled with psychological therapy is commonly used. Hospital based care (e.g., inpatient care, hospitalization, residential care) is needed when an eating disorder leads to extreme physical and medical complications. Treatment may be provided in hospitals, treatment facilities, and office settings. The appropriate form of treatment is decided based on the severity of the eating disorder. Early detection and treatment are beneficial in order to decrease possible medical complications and increase chances of recovery.

DATA AND ANALYSES

Data

Table 26.1 Prevalence of Eating Disorder Symptoms in Males and Females: United States, 2009

Symptom	Males (percentage)	Females (percentage)
Overeating	26.0	18.0
Loss of control over eating	20.0	29.6
Binge eating at least once/week	8.0	10.0
Binge eating at least twice/week	5.8	7.8
Vomiting	1.5	3.7
Fasting	4.0	6.3
Laxative abuse	3.0	3.1
Excessive exercise	5.6	6.0
Body checking	8.9	22.5
Body avoidance	4.4	11.3

Source: DeBar, L., Kraemer, H.C., May, A., Perrin, N., Rosselli, F., Striegel-Moore, R.H., & Wilson, G.T. 2010. "Gender difference in the prevalence of eating disorder symptoms." Retrieved from: http://www.ncbi.nlm.nih.gov/pmc/articles/PMC2696560/

Analysis

Table 26.1 examines the difference in eating disorder symptoms between males and females. Of the respondents for the study, 3,714 were female and 1,808 were male. Data shows that males are more likely to report overeating, while females are more likely to report all other eating disorder symptoms. Similar reports were seen in the symptoms of laxative abuse and excessive exercise; while major differences were seen in the symptoms of overeating, loss of control over eating, body checking, and body avoidance, all of the more prevalent symptoms. Few studies have examined the prevalence of eating disorder symptoms in males. Further research can confirm these statistics and that eating disorders are more prevalent in females.

Data

Table 26.2 Eating Disorders During Adolescence and Psychiatric Conditions During Early Adulthood: United States, 2002

Psychiatric condition	Prevalence among individuals without an eating disorder	Prevalence among individuals with an eating disorder
Anxiety disorder	8%	28%
Depressive disorder	5%	20%
Disruptive disorder	3%	5%
Personality disorder	13%	25%
Substance use disorder	8%	12%
Suicide attempt	3%	12%

Source: Brook, J.S., Cohen, P., Johnson, J.G., & Kasen, S. 2002. "Eating disorders during adolescence and the risk for physical and mental disorders during early adulthood." Retrieved from: http://www.ncbi.nlm.nih.gov/pubmed/12044197

Analysis

Table 26.2 presents the correlation between eating disorder prevalence and additional psychiatric disorders during early adulthood. Anxiety disorders were the most common psychiatric disorders in adolescents with eating disorders at 28%, compared to only 8% of adolescents without eating disorders who presented anxiety disorders. Additionally, there was a high prevalence of depressive disorders among adolescents with eating disorders at 20%, while only 5% of adolescents without eating disorders presented depressive disorders. Furthermore, there were high distinctions between the prevalence of personality disorder and suicide attempts in adolescents with eating disorders. Altogether, adolescents with eating disorders presented a higher prevalence for all psychiatric disorders when compared to adolescents without eating disorders. As a whole, 62% of adolescents with eating disorders presented two or more chronic physical health problems during early adulthood, confirming the severity of eating disorders and what they can lead to. Further research can perform the study on a larger sample to support the findings and examine further connections between eating disorders and co-occurring psychiatric disorders.

Data

Table 26.3 Average Age of Onset and Persistence of Eating Disorders

Type of eating disorder	Average age of onset	Years with episode
Anorexia nervosa	18.9	1.7
Bulimia nervosa	19.7	8.3
Binge-eating disorder	25.4	8.1
Subthreshold binge-eating disorder	22.7	7.2
Any binge-eating	22.4	8.7

Source: Hiripi, E., Hudson, J.I., & Kessler, R.C. 2007. "The prevalence and correlates of eating disorders in the National Comorbidity Survey Replication." Retrieved from: http://www.ncbi.nlm.nih.gov/pmc/articles/PMC1892232/

Analysis

Table 26.3 presents the average age of onset for eating disorders, as well as the persistence based on how many years individuals suffered with the specific eating disorder. Subthreshold binge-eating disorder was defined for the study as binge-eating episodes that occurred at least twice a week for at least three months and occurred solely during the course of anorexia nervosa, bulimia nervosa, or binge-eating disorder. Any binge-eating was defined as binge-eating episodes occurring at least twice a week for at least three months, but lacking the criteria of exhibiting another eating disorder as well. The median age of onset for all five disorders ranged from 18 to 25 years old. Anorexia nervosa presented the earliest average age of onset at 18.9 years old, but also the shortest persistence with an average episode of 1.7 years. Bulimia nervosa's average age of onset followed at 19.7 years old; however, the persistence greatly increased to 8.3 years. Furthermore, binge-eating behaviors tended to appear later between the ages of 22 and 25; however, they also presented persistent episodes that lasted about eight years. Further research can examine the cause of a greater persistence in bulimia nervosa and binge-eating disorders than anorexia nervosa, as well as the cause for the difference in average age of onset.

DISCUSSION QUESTIONS

1. How can eating disorders be detected among males to ensure better accuracy of research? What measures can be taken to encourage individuals suffering from eating disorders to seek treatment?
2. Why does binge-eating disorder have the highest lifetime prevalence? How do society's views on food and physical appearance relate to the prevalence of eating disorders?
3. What are the crude mortality rates for binge-eating disorder, other specified eating disorders, and nonspecified eating disorders?
4. What measures can be taken to reduce the number of suicides attempted by individuals suffering from eating disorders?
5. What measures can be taken before the average ages of onset for eating disorders in order to prevent the development of these disorders? At what age should educational information and healthy body image discussions be introduced to children to help prevent them from developing these disorders?

27

EXERCISE/PHYSICAL ACTIVITY

INTRODUCTION

Understanding Exercise and Physical Activity

Aside from maintaining a balanced diet, exercising and being physically active are essential to leading a healthy life. In fact, without them an individual is more at risk for certain diseases, illnesses, and conditions.

Physical activity refers to anything that keeps a person's body moving, regardless of what, how, when, or where. It is usually categorized into aerobic activity ("cardio"), which increases heart rate and breathing, muscle-strengthening activity, which help work on the muscle groups of the body, bone-strengthening activity, which make bones more resilient, or balance and stretching activity, which are important for the body's stability. There are countless activities in each category, as well as a variety of intensities from light, moderate, to vigorous that indicate to what degree the body is exercising or exerting energy.

Some examples from both categories of physical activity include:

- Walking, hiking, jogging, running
- Riding a bike
- Playing a sport
- Swimming
- Doing push-ups, pull-ups, and sit-ups
- Dancing
- Gardening
- Climbing stairs
- Lifting weights
- Yoga

Guidelines

When it comes to exercise and physical activity, there are several different guidelines for people in different age groups. According to the *2008 Physical Activity Guidelines for Americans,* (U.S. Department of Health and Human Services, 2008), adults should either get at least 150 minutes of moderate-intensity physical activity, 75 minutes of vigorous-intensity activity, or an equivalent mix of both. Children should participate in at least 60 minutes of physical activity daily.

Benefits

Many people consider exercise a hobby because they enjoy being physically active, but it is more than just a fun activity—it also has plenty of benefits for the mind and body. These advantages are indiscriminate and can be enjoyed by all individuals, regardless of their age, ethnicity, or weight. Some of the main benefits of exercise and physical activity include:

- Help maintain or lose weight
- Reduce risk for cardiac events and cardiovascular disease
- Reduce risk for type 2 diabetes and metabolic syndrome
- Reduce risk for colon and breast cancers
- Improve sleep
- Slow down the loss of bone density

- Strengthen and build bones, muscles, and joints
- Relieve stress
- Improve mental health and mood
- Prevent falls
- Increases lifespan

DATA AND ANALYSES

Data

Table 27.1 Percentage of U.S. Youth Aged 12–15 Years Who Were Physically Active Daily, by Sex and Weight Status, 2012

Sex/weight status	Percentage
Boys	
Normal weight	29.5
Overweight	29.5
Obese	18.0
Girls	
Normal weight	24.1
Overweight	20.1
Obese	19.6

Note: In this table data, physically active is defined as engaging in moderate to vigorous physical activity.

Source: Tala, F., Hughes, J., Burt, V. L., MinKyoung, S., Fulton, J.E. and Ogden, C.L., Physical Activity in U.S. Youth Aged 12–15 Years, 2012, NCHS Data Brief No. 141, Jan. 2014. Retrieved from: http://www.cdc.gov/nchs/data/databriefs/db141_table.pdf#1

Analysis

Table 27.1 demonstrates the percentage of U.S. boys and girls between the ages of 12 and 15 who were considered physically active daily in 2012. This data classified the boys and girls into three weight statuses: normal weight, overweight, and obese.

For girls, a greater weight translated into a lower percentage— or a fewer number of girls participating in moderate to vigorous physical activity daily. For example, there were 24.1% active normal-weight girls, 20.1% active overweight girls, and 19.6% active obese girls.

Likewise, obese boys held the lowest percentage out of the male weight statuses, 18.0%. Interesting, the percentage for normal-weight and overweight boys was the same, 29.5%.

Data

Table 27.2 Percentage of Participation in Leisure-time Aerobic and Muscle-strengthening Activities that Meet 2008 *Physical Activity Guidelines for Americans* Among Adults Aged 18 and Over, Selected Years Between 1998 and 2012

	Percent meeting both aerobic and muscle-strengthening guidelines		Percent meeting neither aerobic nor muscle-strengthening guidelines	
	1998	2012	1998	2012
18–24 years old	23.8	29.7	46.5	37.9
25–44 years old	17.4	24.2	51.9	42.2
45–54 years old	13.2	18.2	56.9	48.3
55–64 years old	8.6	16.0	61.8	51.2
65–74 years old	7.0	14.8	65.6	51.7
≥75 years old	3.5	7.9	77.8	67.2
Total ≥18 years old, Age-adjusted	14.3	20.8	56.6	46.6

Source: http://www.cdc.gov/nchs/data/hus/2013/068.pdf

Analysis

Table 27.2 shows the change in participation in aerobic and muscle-strengthening activities that met the *2008 Physical Activity Guidelines* for adults 18 years and older. The data takes into account two years more than a decade apart—1998 and 2012.

In 2012, there was a higher total percentage of adults 18 years or older who met physical activity guidelines for aerobic and muscle-strengthening activities. In the same year, there was a lower percentage of adults 18 years and older who did not meet physical activity guidelines for aerobic and muscle-strengthening activities.

These relationships were mirrored by the individual percentages of every age group in the data table. Every age range in general showed that more people were meeting the *2008 Physical Activity Guidelines* in 2012 than they were in 1998.

It is also worth mentioning that in both 1998 and 2012, each percentage for those meeting the guidelines decreased with increasing age—that is, the older the age group, the harder it was for that age group to meet the guidelines. For those who did not meet either of the guidelines, the reverse was true. The percentages, with the exception of the 75-and-older age group, increased with each consecutive age range.

Data

Table 27.3 Percentage of U.S. Adults Aged 18 and Over Whose Physician or Other Health Professional Recommended Exercise or Physical Activity by Sex and Year, 2000, 2005, and 2010

Sex/year	Percentage
Men	
2000	21.0
2005	27.1
2010	30.3
Women	
2000	23.9
2005	31.2
2010	34.1
Total	
2000	22.6
2005	29.4
2010	32.4

Note: Data takes into account adults aged 18 and over who had seen a physician or other health professional in the past 12 months.

Source: Barnes, Patricia and Schoenborn, Trends in Adults Receiving a Recommendation for Exercise or Other Physical Activity from a Physician or Other Health Professional, NCHS Data Brief No. 86, Feb. 2012. Retrieved from: http://www.cdc.gov/nchs/data/databriefs/db86_fig1.png

Analysis

Table 27.3 shows the percentage of U.S. adults 18 years and older whose doctors recommended some form of exercise or physical activity in 2000, 2005, and 2010. For men, woman, and both sexes combined, the trend in numbers was the same—with each consecutive year, a higher percentage of patients was being recommended exercise and physical activity by their doctors. For example, 22.6% of men and women were given the suggestion by their health care professionals in 2000, while 32.4% of them were given the same a decade later in 2010.

DISCUSSION QUESTIONS

1. Exercise and physical activity can be extremely advantageous to individuals, whether or not they have health problems.

Can you name some of the benefits of exercising and being active, aside from those listed above?

2. You might have heard of the saying, "Everything in moderation." Do you think this phrase applies to exercise and physical activity? Is there such thing as getting *too much* exercise, and if so, what can happen to an individual?

3. In 2012, there was a higher total percentage of adults 18 years or older who met physical activity guidelines for aerobic and muscle-strengthening activities than there were in 1998. What are some possible reasons for this change?

4. Most physically inactive individuals cannot begin exercising with vigorous-intensity aerobic activities. Using the list of activity types above, how would you suggest for someone to build up to this intensity over time?

5. According to the data above, a higher percentage of normal-weight boys and girls are physically active daily than obese boys and girls are. Considering physical and emotional components, why might it be more difficult for obese boys and girls to exercise and participate in physical activity?

28

FOOD-BORNE ILLNESSES

INTRODUCTION

Understanding Food-borne Illnesses

Food-borne illnesses, also commonly referred to as food poisoning, are caused by disease-causing microbes, pathogens, poisonous chemicals, and other harmful substances that contaminate foods or beverages. Over 250 different food-borne illnesses have been identified, most classified as infections that are caused by food-borne bacteria, viruses, and parasites, while fewer are classified as poisonings caused by chemicals or toxic substances.

While the majority of individuals with food-borne illnesses will often recover on their own without seeking any medical attention, food-borne illnesses can lead to severe complications and even be fatal. Understanding and preventing food-borne illnesses is a serious matter, as they can lead to outbreaks where a group of people consume the same contaminated food and all are infected, yet many remain localized, identified, and controlled.

Food-borne illnesses reach humans various ways, as there are multiple processes that go into preparing many of the foods that Americans eat. Often, food-borne pathogens are already present in healthy animals that are raised for food, but contamination can also occur during the slaughtering of animals. Fruits and vegetables can become contaminated if they are washed by unsanitary water that is infected by animal manure or human sewage. Additionally, oysters, shellfish, and other foods that come from the ocean can be contaminated by human sewage that is dumped in the sea. In each case, the harmful toxins contaminate the food before humans receive it; however, contamination can also occur because of unsanitary preparation conditions, such as not washing one's hands or cross-contaminating raw foods.

Symptoms

Symptoms of food-borne illnesses may not appear for hours or days after ingesting contaminated food, depending on the incubation period of the pathogen and the amount that was ingested. During the incubation period, the illness-causing organism attaches to the walls of the intestines and multiplies until it is absorbed into the bloodstream or directly invades body tissues. Symptoms of food-borne illnesses then become apparent; however, various symptoms may be experienced since each food-borne illness is caused by a different infectious or poisonous substance. Since the harmful toxins enter the body through the gastrointestinal tract, many initial and common symptoms of food-borne illnesses include:

- Nausea
- Vomiting
- Abdominal cramps
- Diarrhea
- Fever

The initial symptoms listed above may lead to more severe symptoms, such as blood in the stool or dehydration, which can be recognized by a decrease in urination, a dry mouth and/or throat, and dizziness.

Diagnosis

It is difficult to diagnose the cause of food-borne illnesses without laboratory tests, since many symptoms overlap. Additionally, the only way to determine the exact cause of food-borne illnesses are through specific laboratory tests. Culturing stool samples often identifies bacterial causes of food-borne illnesses, such as Campylobacter, Salmonella, and E. coli O157. Parasitic causes are found by examining stools under a microscope, while viral causes are harder to identify. Since viruses are too small to detect with a microscope, stool samples are often tested for genetic markers that indicate whether a specific virus is present. Additional experimental tests may be used to identify causes of food-borne illnesses; however, these tests can be costly. Therefore, many medical professionals do not run laboratory tests to identify the cause of food-borne illnesses. Many individuals who ingest contaminated food also do not seek medical attention since symptoms usually alleviate on their own within two to three days. For these reasons, many cases of food-borne illnesses go undiagnosed or are not confirmed by laboratory tests.

While medical attention is not required to treat food-borne illnesses, individuals should consult a doctor if they experience a high fever over 101.5 degrees Fahrenheit, blood in the stool, prolonged vomiting, signs of dehydration, or symptoms that last for more than three days. These more serious symptoms may indicate complications from the food-borne illness.

Risk Factors

Certain foods are associated with food-borne illnesses more than others. These foods include raw animal foods, such as meat, poultry, eggs, shellfish, and unpasteurized milk. Additionally, bulk animal products pose an even greater risk of contamination, as a single infected food could potentially contaminate the entire group. Fruits and vegetables also pose a high risk of contamination, as they must be thoroughly washed to decrease chances of contamination.

Unsanitary food preparation also greatly increases the risk of contracting food-borne illnesses. Cross contamination may occur if foods are transferred with the same knife, cutting board, or other kitchen utensil as a contaminated food. Therefore, it is important to wash these utensils and surfaces when preparing food, as fully cooked food can also become recontaminated by touching other raw foods or contaminated surfaces. Additionally, food should not be left out, as warm, moist conditions allows bacteria to grow and reproduce to certain contamination levels that otherwise would cause no harm. Storing food in the refrigerator or freezer will help to prevent contamination. When cooking, it is important for individuals to wash their hands. In addition, raw animal products should be cooked with high heat, which often kills harmful pathogens. It is recommended that raw animal products should be cooked until internal temperatures are above 160 degrees Fahrenheit. When preserving foods, it is important to understand that high salt, sugar, and acidity levels help prevent bacteria from growing.

Specific populations are also more vulnerable to food-borne illnesses, including pregnant females, the elderly, and other individuals with weakened immune systems. Bottle-fed infants are also at a high risk of developing food-borne illnesses, especially if the baby formula is left at room temperature. Additionally, individuals with liver disease are more susceptible to food-borne illnesses; however, they typically only pose a higher risk for a single pathogen found in oysters.

Treatment

Treatment for food-borne illnesses often depends on the severity of symptoms and cause. In most cases, symptoms from food-borne illnesses will resolve on their own within two to three days, so medical attention is not required. Many medical professionals will not provide antibiotics for food-borne illnesses, as they do not want individuals to build up a resistance to the antibiotic; in any case, viral-caused food-borne illnesses would not respond to the antibiotic.

However, individuals who primarily experience the symptoms of diarrhea and vomiting should be aware of dehydration. If they lose more body fluids and electrolytes than they are ingesting, they may experience the symptoms of dehydration. To keep hydrated, oral rehydration solutions such as Ceralyte, Pedialyte, or Oralyte may be used. Additionally, bismuth subsalicylate solutions, such as Pepto-Bismol, may reduce the duration and severity of symptoms. Antidiarrheal medication may provide relief as well, yet these medications should not be taken if diarrhea and cramps are accompanied by blood in the stool or a fever. In these cases that pose more severe symptoms, antidiarrheal medication may make conditions worse.

DATA AND ANALYSES

Data

Table 28.1 Pathogens Causing the Most Food-borne Illnesses, Hospitalizations, and Deaths Each Year: United States, 2011

Pathogen	Estimated number of illnesses	Estimated number of hospitalizations	Estimated number of deaths
Norovirus	5,461,731	14,663	149
Salmonella, nontyphoidal	1,027,561	19,336	378

Pathogen	Estimated number of illnesses	Estimated number of hospitalizations	Estimated number of deaths
Clostridium perfringens	965,958	438	26
Campylobacter spp.	845,024	8,463	76
Staphylococcus aureus	241,148	1,064	6
Toxoplasma gondii	86,686	4,428	327
E. coli (STEC) O157	63,153	2,138	20
Listeria monocytogenes	1,591	1,455	255
Subtotal	8,693,022	51,985	1,237

Source: Centers for Disease Control and Prevention. 2014. "CDC estimates of foodborne illness in the United States." Retrieved from: http://www.cdc.gov/foodborneburden/resources.html#estimate_tables

Analysis

Table 28.1 presents the pathogens that cause the most food-borne illnesses, hospitalizations, and deaths each year in the United States. The four most common food-borne illnesses are: norovirus, which is the most common and spreads from person to person via contaminated food, water or environmental surfaces rather than animals; Salmonella, which originates in the intestines of birds, reptiles, and mammals; Clostridium perfringens, which is most commonly found in raw meat and poultry; and Campylobacter, which originates in the intestines of birds and raw meat. Campylobacter is also the bacterial pathogen that is responsible for the most bacterial-caused diarrheal illnesses in the world.

Altogether, the eight common pathogens result in over 8.5 million food-borne illnesses per year, over 50,000 of which lead to hospitalizations and over 1,200 of which lead to death. The pathogens that cause the most illnesses and hospitalizations are relatively similar; however, the death-causing pathogens do not correlate. Besides norovirus and Salmonella, both of which are the leading causes of food-borne illnesses each year, Toxoplasma gondii and Listeria monocytogenes also present as the top causes of food-borne-illness-related deaths. Further research can determine why the two less common pathogens contribute to so many deaths and how they can be detected and prevented.

Data

Table 28.2 Changes in Incidences of Laboratory Confirmed Bacterial-caused Food-borne Illnesses: United States, 2013 Incidences Compared to 2010–2012 Incidences

Pathogen	Decrease/increase
Campylobacter spp.	2% increase
Listeria monocytogenes	3% decrease
Salmonella, nontyphoidal	9% decrease
Shigella spp.	14% increase
E. coli (STEC) Non-O157	8% increase
E. coli (STEC) O157	16% increase
Vibrio spp.	32% increase
Yersinia enterocolitica	7% increase

Source: National Center for Emerging and Zoonotic Infectious Diseases and Division of Foodborne, Waterborne and Environmental diseases. 2014. "Trends in foodborne illness in the United States, 2013." Centers for Disease Control and Prevention. Retrieved from: http://www.cdc.gov/features/dsfoodsafetyreport/

Analysis

Table 28.2 examines the prevalence of bacterial-caused food-borne illnesses in the United States, comparing incidences from the year 2013 to incidences that occurred between the years 2010 and 2012. Listeria monocytogenes presented a 3% decrease, alongside Salmonella, which decreased 9%; however, when compared to the longer term baseline that examined 2006 and 2008 incidences, Salmonella rates remained the same. All other bacterial-caused food-borne illnesses posed an increase in incidence rates.

Campylobacter spp. infections only rose 2% between 2010 and 2013; however, overall rates have increased 13% since the 2006–2008 period. E. coli, Shigella, and Yersinia enterocolitica rates have all increased between 2010 and 2013, with no additional significant increase when examining 2006–2008 incidences. Most significantly, Vibrio infections increased 32% between 2010 and 2013, now at the highest incidence rates since their original tracking in 1996. Further research can examine why bacterial-caused food-borne illnesses are increasing over the years and how these incidences can start to be decreased.

DISCUSSION QUESTIONS

1. How do food-borne pathogens spread among animal species? How can this be prevented to lower the amount of contamination that humans ingest?

2. How can individuals ensure that fruits and vegetables are washed with sanitary water after harvesting to prevent contamination?

3. How can individuals ensure that fresh manure used to fertilize vegetables does not cause contamination?

4. Why do Toxoplasma gondii and Listeria monocytogenes present as two of the four most common death-causing pathogens related to food-borne illnesses when they are some of the least common illnesses?

5. Why are bacterial-caused food-borne illnesses increasing? How can these numbers start to be decreased?

29

HIV/AIDS

INTRODUCTION

Understanding HIV/AIDS

One of the most deadly infections that has been plaguing humans exclusively and that has become widespread in the past several decades is the human immunodeficiency virus, commonly known as HIV. This virus, once contracted, attacks key actors in the human immune system like T-cells to make copies of itself before destroying them. Unlike other viruses, however, HIV does not allow a person's immune system to drive it out over time. Instead, the infection weakens the immune system and prevents it from fighting against it and other infections or diseases.

When the HIV infection overpowers the immune system's ability to effectively do its job, it becomes acquired immunodeficiency syndrome, commonly referred to as AIDS. This is considered the final stage of HIV. Not everyone who suffers from HIV contracts AIDS.

Symptoms

Within the first month of an HIV infection, a person begins to exhibit several flu-like symptoms that result as the body's natural response to the HIV infection. The symptoms can last from days to weeks, and even months. However, many of them are symptoms of other conditions, infections, and diseases. Keeping this in mind, the symptoms of a primary HIV infection include:

- Fever
- Swollen lymph glands
- Sore throat
- Rash
- Fatigue
- Muscle aches and pains
- Joint aches and pains
- Headache
- Chills
- Night sweats
- Diarrhea

Once the primary HIV infection passes the clinical latency stage, during which it continues to develop without exhibiting symptoms, it progresses to AIDS. During this very late stage in the infection, symptoms begin to reappear and are more aggressive, but they are still symptoms of other conditions, infections, and diseases. Symptoms of the HIV infection when it transitions to AIDS include:

- Recurring fever
- Rapid weight loss
- Prolonged lymph gland swelling
- Mouth, anus, and genital sores
- Discolored blemishes on skin, mouth, nose, and eyelids
- Fatigue
- Memory loss
- Depression
- Profuse night sweats
- Diarrhea lasting longer than one week

Diagnosis

Although the aforementioned symptoms are strong indicators of HIV/AIDS, they are not given full consideration by whoever is making a diagnosis. The only way for a person to know with certainty whether or not they have HIV/AIDS is to get tested.

Testing usually comes in the form of blood, saliva, or urine analysis that checks for HIV antibodies. Unfortunately, the body can take anywhere from three to six months to produce these antibodies, which stalls early detection. Moreover, results from the most common of these tests, the enzyme immunoassay, can take up to two weeks to return.

The United States Food and Drug Administration, however, recently approved a rapid diagnostic test to detect both early-stage HIV antibodies and HIV antigen, which is a particular protein generated by the virus immediately after infection. The new rapid diagnostic tool allows people diagnosed with HIV to receive proper treatment faster and prevent further transmission of the HIV infection to others.

Once a person is diagnosed with HIV/AIDS, they can undergo other tests to get more details about their infection and tailor treatment to the stage of their infection. For example, they can receive a CD4 count, which determine the number of white blood cells that the HIV infection targets left in their body. If a person's CD4 count is below 200 cells, it signifies AIDS.

Other tests, like viral load and resistance, check blood in a different way to see the amount of HIV in the body and how resistant it will be to certain medications.

Risk Factors

There are many risk factors for HIV/AIDS that are indiscriminate of age or race. Luckily, most of them are preventable for this reason. There is a common misconception that HIV/AIDS can only infect men who engage in intercourse with other men, but it can also infect heterosexual men and women. The risk factors that make contracting HIV/AIDS more likely include:

- Having unprotected vaginal or anal sex
- Having oral sex
- Having multiple sexual partners
- Having a sexually transmitted infection (STI)
- Using intravenous drugs and sharing related intravenous drug paraphernalia with others
- Being an uncircumcised man

Treatment

Unfortunately, there is currently no known cure for HIV/AIDS, but doctors, scientists, and researchers are working to find one. Until then, patients suffering from the infection must rely on treatment in the form of one or more of approximately 30 approved drugs used for antiretroviral therapy. The antiretroviral drugs, which come in the form of orally ingested pills, are all separated into five different classes. Each class signifies how the medication deters HIV replication within the body. In general, patients are prescribed a combination of three medications from two classes.

The key to fighting HIV/AIDS is taking the right combination of antiretroviral medications at the right dosages that will result in the least possible number of short- and long-term side effects. With any and all combinations of HIV/AIDS medications, people diagnosed with the infection can expect to experience:

- Anemia
- Nausea and vomiting
- Headaches
- Dizziness
- Pain and nerve problems
- Lipodystrophy, or fat redistribution
- Insulin resistance
- Lipid abnormalities
- Decrease in bone density
- Lactic acidosis, or a buildup of cell waste in the body

After the HIV infection is exposed to the same medications for extended periods, it typically mutates and becomes immune to them. When this occurs, many people volunteer to take part in clinical trials specifically geared towards HIV/AIDS. During these trials, researchers work with volunteers to see if a new treatment or device can safely prevent or fight HIV.

DATA AND ANALYSES

Data

Table 29.1 Estimated New HIV Infections in the United States for Most Affected Populations, 2010

Population	Number of new HIV infections
White MSM	11,200
Black MSM	10,600
Hispanic/Latino MSM	6,700
Black heterosexual women	5,300
Black heterosexual men	2,700
White heterosexual women	1,300

Population	Number of new HIV infections
Hispanic/Latino heterosexual women	1,200
Black male IDU	1,100
Black female IDU	850

Note: Subpopulations representing <2% of the epidemic are not reflected. "MSM" denotes men who have sex with men, while "IDU" denotes injection drug users.

Source: HIV in the United States at a Glance, U.S. Statistics, AIDS.gov. Retrieved from: http://aids.gov/hiv-aids-basics/hiv-aids-101/statistics/index.html

Analysis

Table 29.1 provides an overview of the United States populations that contracted an HIV infection in 2010. White and black men who have or have had sex with other men were the two groups with the most significant number of new HIV infections, with 11,200 and 10,600, respectively. Hispanic and Latino men who have or have had sex with other men were close behind with a total of 6,700 new HIV infections before any heterosexual populations—male or female—made the 2010 data.

Homosexual and heterosexual men and women of various races and ethnicities were not the only populations to contract HIV in 2010, however. Injection drug users were also an important population. Interestingly, black male and women were the only groups to represent more than 2% of the overall epidemic.

Data

Table 29.2 Rate of HIV Infection in the United States by Year of Diagnosis and Age, 2008–2011

Age	2008	2009	2010	2011
<13 years old	0.5	0.4	0.4	0.4
13–14 years old	0.5	0.4	0.5	0.6
15–19 years old	10.4	10.4	9.9	10.4
20–24 years old	31.4	32.3	34.4	36.4
25–29 years old	33.0	31.2	31.7	35.2
30–34 years old	32.1	29.7	28.9	30.3
35–39 years old	31.6	28.5	26.8	27.0
40–44 years old	32.6	29.5	26.6	27.4
45–49 years old	26.6	23.7	22.6	25.1

(Continued)

Table 29.2 Rate of HIV Infection in the United States by Year of Diagnosis and Age, 2008–2011 (*Continued*)

Age	2008	2009	2010	2011
50–54 years old	18.2	17.3	16.4	17.5
55–59 years old	12.5	11.6	11.0	11.4
60–64 years old	7.7	6.5	6.6	6.9
≥65 years old	2.4	2.1	2.0	2.3

Note: Rates are per 100,000 population.

Source: Rates of diagnoses of HIV infection among adults and adolescents, by area of residence, 2011—United States and 6 dependent areas, Diagnoses of HIV Infection in the United States and Dependent Areas, 2011 Vol. 23, HIV Surveillance Report. Retrieved from: http://www.cdc.gov/hiv/pdf/statistics_2011_HIV_Surveillance_Report_vol_23.pdf#Page=40

Analysis

Table 29.2 reflects the trends in HIV infection rates in the United States by year of diagnosis and age from 2008 to 2011. For all four years, the rate for children up to 14 years was less than 1.0, and was between 2.0 and 2.5 for adults older than 65 years.

Interestingly, in 2009, 2010, and 2011, the 20–24 age group exhibited the highest rate of HIV infection diagnosis. In 2008, the highest rate was exhibited in the 40–44 age group.

DISCUSSION QUESTIONS

1. Primary HIV infection symptoms are similar to flu symptoms. What other diseases, viruses, or conditions can you name that also have flu-like symptoms?
2. There is a common misconception that HIV/AIDS can only infect men who have sex with other men. What are some possible reasons for this widespread mistaken belief? Using what you now know about HIV/AIDS risk factors, why is it wrong?
3. Not everyone who suffers from an HIV infection gets AIDS. How is this possible?
4. Currently, there is no known cure for HIV/AIDS, but researchers are constantly working to find one. Considering any problems or lack of resources researchers might encounter, why do you think finding a cure has proved so difficult?
5. Several tests can be conducted on a person once they find out they have HIV/AIDS for more details on their infection. How might a resistance test be able to check what medications will or will not work in treating the infection?

30

HYPERTENSION

INTRODUCTION

Understanding Hypertension

As a principal vital sign, blood pressure is an important aspect of health that must be monitored frequently and kept under control at all times. Luckily, blood pressure is quickly, easily, and painlessly measured using an inflatable arm cuff and pressure gauge that together provide a ratio of systolic to diastolic numbers in millimeters of mercury—that is, a ratio of the pressure in any given artery during heartbeats over the pressure between them in millimeters of mercury (mmHg). An example of a normal blood pressure reading would be any ratio of systolic and diastolic numbers under 120/80 mmHg.

When the force of blood flowing through a person's blood vessels surpasses this ratio and reaches such an abnormally high level that it begins to cause serious problems within the body, a person suffers from high blood pressure, or hypertension. In people under 60 years of age, a 140/90 mmHg pressure read is considered hypertensive. In people over 60 years of age, this pressure ratio changes to 150/90 mmHg.

Diagnosis

Hypertension is sometimes referred to as the "silent killer" by medical professionals because of a lack of symptoms that makes it difficult for people to realize they have the condition. This uncertainty is what makes high blood pressure unlike other conditions, which usually have a clear-cut, defined set of warning signs that make it easy for doctors and nurses to make a diagnosis.

Because hypertension patients cannot rely on symptoms to indicate a problem, the only way to know whether or not they have high blood pressure is to get their blood pressure levels checked with an inflatable arm cuff at home, at a doctor's office, or even in some stores.

Risk Factors

Generally, hypertension risk factors can be categorized into heredity, preexisting conditions, and lifestyle behaviors. The most common risk factors in these categories include:

- Family history of high blood pressure
- Prehypertension
- Diabetes
- Chronic kidney disease
- Obesity
- Old age
- Diets high in sodium, cholesterol, and saturated or total fat
- Smoking
- Drinking alcohol to excess
- Physical inactivity

Although some risk factors like family history cannot be controlled, most others can be addressed, controlled, or minimized by hypertension patients if they make gradual changes to their lifestyles.

Effects

Mainly targeting the circulatory system, hypertension can negatively affect different organs of the body, including the brain, eyes, kidneys, and heart, as well as major arteries. These effects include but are not limited to:

- Stroke
- Burst eye vessels
- Impaired vision
- Aneurysms

- Heart attack
- Congestive heart failure
- Angina
- Kidney failure
- Dizziness
- Narrowing of arteries

Treatment

Once a patient is diagnosed with hypertension, treatment can begin on two fronts—lifestyle choices and medications. To combat any increase in blood pressure, a person can take initiative and on their own stop smoking, drinking excessive amounts of alcohol, and eating foods with sodium, cholesterol, and fat. Instead, they are encouraged to be physically active, manage their weight, and reduce stress.

Along with these lifestyle changes, there are hundreds of special medications that hypertension patients can take to get their blood pressure levels back to normal. The most common are diuretics or "water pills," which work with the kidneys to remove water and salt from the body, gradually reducing the amount of fluid in the blood that flows through the arteries and therefore reducing the blood pressure of the patient's body.

Other medicinal options to bring blood pressure levels back down to normal include beta-blockers, alpha-blockers, and angio-tensin-converting enzyme (ACE) inhibitors. While beta-blockers slow down the blood-pumping activity of the heart and allow blood to flow with considerably less force through the arteries, alpha-blockers relax blood vessels by controlling nerve impulses. On the other hand, ACE inhibitors reduce the production of the angiotensin II hormone that tightens blood vessels, making them more relaxed for blood to flow more freely and with less pressure.

DATA AND ANALYSES

Data

Table 30.1 Hypertension Prevalence Among U.S. Adults Aged 18 and Over, Age-specific and Age-adjusted, 2011–2012

	Percentage affected
Sex	
Men	29.7%
Women	28.5%

(Continued)

Table 30.1 Hypertension Prevalence Among U.S. Adults Aged 18 and Over, Age-specific and Age-adjusted, 2011–2012 (*Continued*)

	Percentage affected
Age	
18–39 years old	7.3%
40–59 years old	32.4%
60 years and older	65.0%
Race and ethnicity	
Non-Hispanic white	28.0%
Non-Hispanic black	42.1%
Non-Hispanic Asian	24.7%
Hispanic	26.0%
Overall	**29.1%**

Note: Data is age-specific and age-adjusted.

Source: http://www.cdc.gov/nchs/data/databriefs/db133.htm

Analysis

Taking into account sex, age, race, and ethnicity provides valuable insight into exactly who is affected by hypertension. Table 30.1 includes these specific categories of data to identify Americans over 18 with hypertension from 2011 to 2012. During this time frame, the Centers for Disease Control and Prevention found that 29.1% of Americans overall suffer from high blood pressure. Although the sex of a person does not have a considerable impact on the numbers, age, race, and ethnicity do.

When considering age, the table data shows that the older a person is, the more susceptible they are to hypertension. In fact, the age numbers show a significant linear trend, with only 7.3% of people affected in the 18–39 age group, 32.4% in the 40–59 age group, and 65.0% in the 60-and-older age group. The percentage of those affected in the oldest age range is approximately nine times that of the youngest age range.

When considering race and ethnicity, 28.0% of Non-Hispanic whites, 24.7% of Non-Hispanic Asians, and 26.0% of Hispanics were affected by hypertension. Although these three groups had percentages within 5% of each other, they were all significantly lower than Non-Hispanic blacks, of which 42.1%—the highest of all races and ethnicities—were affected by high blood pressure.

Data

Table 30.2 Number, Percentage, and Percent Change of Leading Causes of Death in the United States, 2010

Rank	Number of total deaths	Percent of total deaths	Percent change from 2009 to 2010
All causes of death	2,468,435	100%	−0.3%
Diseases of heart	597,689	24.2%	−2.0%
Malignant neoplasms	574,743	23.3%	−0.4%
Chronic lower respiratory diseases	138,080	5.6%	−1.2%
Cerebrovascular diseases	129,476	5.2%	−1.3%
Accidents and unintentional injuries	120,859	4.9%	1.3%
Alzheimer's disease	83,494	3.4%	3.7%
Diabetes mellitus	69,071	2.8%	−1.0%
Nephritis, nephrotic syndrome, and nephrosis	50,476	2.0%	1.3%
Influenza and pneumonia	50,097	2.0%	−8.5%
Intentional self-harm and suicide	38,364	1.6%	2.5%
Septicemia	34,812	1.4%	−3.6%
Chronic liver disease and cirrhosis	31,903	1.3%	3.3%
Essential hypertension and hypertensive renal disease	26,634	1.1%	2.6%
Parkinson's disease	22,032	0.9%	4.6%
Pneumonitis due to solids and liquids	17,011	0.7%	4.1%

Note: Only data showing percent-change from 2009 to 2010 is age-adjusted.

Source: http://www.cdc.gov/nchs/data/nvsr/nvsr61/nvsr61_04.pdf

Analysis

Data from the Centers for Disease Control and Prevention in Table 30.2 shows the 15 leading causes of death in the United States in 2010. During this specific year, essential hypertension and hypertensive renal disease was the 13th leading cause of death, fatally affecting 26,634 people and ranking just above Parkinson's disease and pneumonitis due to solids and liquids.

Although essential hypertension and hypertensive renal disease accounted for a relatively small percentage of deaths (1.1%)

compared to causes of death higher up in the chart like heart disease (24.2%), this category actually showed the fifth largest age-adjusted increase from 2009 to 2010, rising 2.6% from the former year, following close behind other categories like Parkinson's disease at 4.6%, pneumonitis at 4.1%, Alzheimer's disease at 3.7%, and chronic liver disease and cirrhosis at 3.3%.

It is also worth noting that because hypertension increases the risk of heart disease and cerebrovascular diseases like stroke, it can be directly linked to many of the deaths in the first and fourth categories—heart disease (24.2%) and cerebrovascular diseases (5.2%), respectively.

DISCUSSION QUESTIONS

1. People suffering from hypertension are usually subject to heart disease and cerebrovascular diseases like stroke. What aspects of high blood pressure might increase a person's risk for contracting these other conditions?
2. The data above shows that older Americans are most susceptible to hypertension. What differentiates people in the 18–39 age group from those in the 40-and-older age range?
3. Hypertension, although a seemingly minor category in comparison to other conditions, is still considered a leading cause of death in the United States and is often referred to by medical professionals as the "silent killer." How or in what way might hypertension become fatal if it is left untreated?
4. One of the risk factors of hypertension is keeping a diet high in sodium levels. What kind of foods would constitute a healthy eating plan for hypertensive patients?
5. Applying what you know about hypertension, what effect do you think the opposite—low blood pressure—would have on the functioning of the human body?

31

INFANT MORTALITY

INTRODUCTION

Understanding Infant Mortality

Each year, about 25,000 infants die in the United States. Infant mortality refers to the death of a baby before their first birthday. The infant mortality rate, an estimate of the number of deaths for every 1,000 live births, is often used as a measure of a nation's health and well-being.

For every 1,000 babies that are born, six die during their first year of life. The top five leading causes of infant mortality include:

- Infants with serious birth defects
- Infants born preterm before 37 weeks gestation (full term is 40 weeks)
- Infants that are victims of sudden infant death syndrome (SIDS)
- Infants that are affected by maternal complications during pregnancy
- Infants that are victims of injuries

Infant mortality is classified in to three groups: perinatal mortality, including late fetal death from 22 weeks gestation to birth or the death of a newborn up to one week after delivery; neonatal mortality, including newborn deaths occurring within 28 days after birth; and post-neonatal mortality, including the death of infants aged 29 days to one year old.

Symptoms

Some medical conditions and symptoms that females experience during the duration of their pregnancy may have a serious affect on the infant. Pregnant females should be aware of these conditions and symptoms:

- Anemia, which results in fatigue; urinary tract infections, which result in pain or burning when urinating, frequent urges to urinate, nausea, back pain, and urine with an unusual smell or color
- Mental health conditions, which result in the loss of interest in activities and changes in appetite, sleep, and energy levels
- Hypertension
- Gestational diabetes mellitus; and hyperemesis gravidarum, which results in severe nausea and vomiting

Pregnant females should also be aware of symptoms of preterm labor, which could result in the death of an infant. The symptoms occur before 37-weeks' gestation and include:

- Contractions every ten minutes or less
- Change in vaginal discharge
- Pelvic pressure
- Low, dull backache
- Cramps
- Diarrhea

If born preterm, infants may exhibit the following symptoms:

- Breathing problems
- Feeding problems
- Jaundice
- Cerebral palsy
- Developmental delay
- Vision problems
- Hearing problems

Diagnosis

Routine health care check-ups are important throughout the duration of the pregnancy in order to ensure the health of both the mother and the infant. Diagnosis of birth defects and affects due to maternal complications depend on the symptoms presented by the infant. Both regular term and preterm infants can be diagnosed with low birth weight if they weigh less than five pounds, eight ounces at birth. Preterm labor can be diagnosed with various tests if a pregnant women is experiencing regular contractions and the cervix has begun to dilate before 37-weeks' gestation. Tests to determine preterm labor include pelvis exams, ultrasounds, uterine monitoring, fetal monitoring, lab tests, or maturity amniocentesis. Additionally, for a doctor to determine the cause of SIDS, a thorough investigation must be completed, as well as an extensive review of the infant's medical history. Poisoning, metabolic disorders, hyper- or hypothermia, neglect, homicide, and suffocation are all causes of SIDS.

Risk Factors

Each of the medical conditions that can appear during pregnancy listed above pose higher risks for infant mortality. A primary determinant of infant mortality is infant birth weight, as lower birth weights increase the risk of death. Determinants of low birth weight include economic, psychological, behavioral, and environmental factors. Such risk factors include: poor maternal nutrition, lack of prenatal care, maternal sickness during pregnancy, and very commonly, preterm births.

Preterm births, which account for the most infant deaths, pose additional risk factors. Pregnant females pose a greater risk of having a preterm birth if they had a previous preterm birth, are carrying more than one baby, have problems with the uterus or cervix, have chronic health problems or infections, or use drugs during pregnancy. Race is also a risk factor for preterm births, as black females are about 50% more likely than white females to have a preterm birth. Race is also a risk factor for SIDS, as non-Hispanic black and American Indian/Alaska Native infants experience much higher rates of SIDS.

Additionally, several factors of pregnant females can result in a greater risk of birth defects. These include: diet and nutrition, as a lack of folic acid can result in major birth defects of the infant's brain and spine; consumption of alcohol, as the alcohol passes directly to the infant through the placenta and can result in fetal alcohol spectrum disorder; smoking cigarettes and using other drugs, as drug use can result in premature births, birth defects such as cleft lips, and even infant death; vaccinations, as pregnant women are more susceptible to contracting infections that can be passed on to the infant; and lack of health care, as seeking routine trips to the doctor can help prevent any complications during pregnancy.

Treatment

Infants should only be taken home if they can breathe without support, maintain a stable body temperature, breast- or bottle-feed, and steadily gain weight.

Similar to diagnosis, treatment for affects of maternal complications during pregnancy and birth defects varies based on the symptoms presented by the infant. Treatment for low birth weight depends on the situation of the infant and the mother. Infants with low birth weight often must remain in the hospital until they gain weight, while infants that develop additional complications must remain in the hospital for even longer. Commonly, infants are kept in the neonatal intensive care unit (NICU), which holds them in temperature-controlled incubators and uses special feeding techniques. Whenever possible, even infants with low birth weight should be fed their mother's breast milk. Preterm infants are also held in the NICU, where they are placed in incubators, have their vital signs monitored, and fed breast milk and other fluids through a IV feeding tube. Infants that present jaundice may be placed under bilirubin lights to help the liver break down the excess of bilirubin. Some preterm infants may require a blood transfusion if they cannot produce their own red blood cells. Additionally, medication can be administered to help preterm infants mature, develop a stronger heart rate, reduce infection, and increase urine output. In certain cases, surgery may also be used to aid feeding problems, reverse abnormal blood vessel development and limit further risks to vision, and to drain excess fluid in the brain.

DATA AND ANALYSES

Data

Table 31.1 Infant, Neonatal, and Post-neonatal Mortality Rates, by Race/Ethnicity: United States, 2009

Race/ethnicity	Neonatal mortality rates per 1,000 live births	Post-neonatal mortality rates per 1,000 live births	Infant mortality rates per 1,000 live births
Non-Hispanic white	3.40	1.93	5.33
Non-Hispanic black	8.13	4.27	12.40
American Indian/ Alaska Native	4.38	4.09	8.47
Asian/Pacific Islander	3.11	1.29	4.40
Hispanic	3.56	1.73	5.29
Mexican	3.44	1.67	5.12
Puerto Rican	4.76	2.42	7.18
Cuban	3.61	2.10	5.77
Central and South American	3.17	1.30	4.47
Average total	4.18	2.21	6.39

Source: MacDorman, M.F., & Mathews, T.J. 2013. "Infant mortality statistics from the 2009 period linked birth/infant death data set." Centers for Disease Control and Prevention. Retrieved from: http://www.cdc.gov/nchs/data/nvsr/nvsr61/nvsr61_08.pdf

Analysis

Table 31.1 examines infant mortality categorized by race/ethnicity and age of the infant. The neonatal infant mortality rate includes infants under 28 days old, the post-neonatal infant mortality rate includes infants between 28 days old and one-year-old, and infant mortality rates include all infants under one-year-old. The infant mortality deaths were weighted, which is why some neonatal and post-neonatal mortality rates did not exactly add up to the total infant mortality rate.

Currently, about two-thirds of infant deaths in the United States occur during the neonatal period, while the rest occur during the post-neonatal period. The data table examined these deaths based on race/ethnicity. Results show that the highest infant mortality rate occurred among non-Hispanic black infants, which was more than double the infant mortality rate of non-Hispanic white infants. American Indian/Alaska Native and Puerto Rican infants also presented high infant mortality rates, while the other race/ethnicity groups posed slightly lower, similar rates.

Neonatal infant mortality rates were also highest among non-Hispanic black infants, followed by Puerto Rican and American Indian/Alaska Native infants. Post-neonatal infant mortality followed the same trend, with non-Hispanic black infants and American Indian/Alaska Native infant rates more than doubling the mortality rates of non-Hispanic white infants. Many of these gaps between infant mortality rates can be explained by preterm births, SIDS, congenital malformations, and injuries. Specifically, neonatal infant mortality rates most commonly relate to preterm births and low birth weight, while post-neonatal infant mortality rates relate to SIDS, congenital malformations, and unintentional injuries.

Data

Table 31.2 Infant Mortality Rates for the Five Leading Causes of Infant Death: United States, 2005 vs. 2009

Cause of infant death	2005 death rate per 100,000 live births	2009 death rate per 100,000 live births
Congenital malformations	134.6	129.7
Short gestation and low birth weight	113.5	109.6
Sudden infant death syndrome	54.0	54.0
Maternal complications	42.7	39.1
Unintentional injuries	26.2	28.4

Source: MacDorman, M.F., & Mathews, T.J. 2013. "Infant mortality statistics from the 2009 period linked birth/infant death data set." Centers for Disease Control and Prevention. Retrieved from: http://www.cdc.gov/nchs/data/nvsr/nvsr61/nvsr61_08.pdf

Analysis

Accounting for 20% of all infant deaths, the leading cause of infant death in the United States during 2009 was congenital malformations, deformations, and chromosomal abnormalities. Following this cause was preterm births and low birth weight, which accounted for 17% of all infant deaths. Subsequently, SIDS accounted for 8% of infant deaths, maternal complications during pregnancy accounted for 6% of infant deaths, and unintentional injuries accounted for 4% of infant deaths. These top five causes of infant mortality were the same in 2008 and 2007. The five causes accounted for 56% of all infant deaths in the United States in 2009. The greatest reduction in causes of infant mortality were seen in maternal complications during pregnancy, as the related infant deaths decreased 8% between 2005 and 2009. The other causes did not see a significant decrease, and there was even a slight increase in infant deaths caused by unintentional injuries during this time period.

DISCUSSION QUESTIONS

1. Why are infant mortality rates higher in some race/ethnicity groups than others? What social, environmental, psychological, biological, and other factors contribute to these differences?
2. Why do neonatal infant mortality rates account for two-thirds of total infant mortality rates, while post-neonatal rates only account for one-third? How can neonatal infant mortality rates be reduced in order to lessen the total infant mortality rate?
3. What measures can be taken to further decrease the rates of infant mortality related to the top five leading causes?
4. Why did infant mortality rates caused by unintentional injuries pose an increase over the period of 2005–2009? What preventative measures can be taken to educate parents and professionals about providing safe environments for infants?
5. What causes account for the other 44% of infant deaths in the United States? How can these causes be eliminated or reduced in order to decrease the infant mortality rate?

32

LIFE EXPECTANCY

INTRODUCTION

What Does Life Expectancy Mean?

Life expectancy is a statistical estimate of how long someone is going to live, compiled by the Centers for Disease Control's National Center for Health Statistics. This number is based on how old people were when they died in years past, and is broken down by race and sex. Other factors go into this as well, such as predisposition to illness, whether someone smokes or drinks, and mental health. Since these numbers are averages, it is common to find people who live far longer or far shorter than the expectancy predicts.

The average life expectancy tends to differ between races and genders, often for scientifically verifiable reasons. For instance, Asian Americans tend to have lower body mass indexes, lower blood glucose, and don't smoke as much, leading to longer lives for this group. Whites tend to have the lowest blood pressure while African Americans tend to have the highest, especially those in the rural South. Low-income African American women and Native American men tend to have the highest rates of obesity.

Having unhealthy blood pressure takes 1.5 years off your average life span, while obesity takes 1.3 years, high blood glucose takes an average of 0.4 years, and smoking takes about 2.1 years. Refraining from smoking and keeping the other three factors at healthy ranges will supposedly increase the expected length of one's life.

How to Increase Life Expectancy

Having a strong body and mind are important for both short- and long-term health. Not only will this decrease your risk of diseases, this will extend your life expectancy.

Exercise is a crucial component in any aspect of one's health. Even low-impact activities like a brisk half-hour walk three times a week increases your heart strength, lung capacity, muscle tone, and flexibility. Lifting weights also contributes to muscle and aerobic strength, as well as increases bone density, a very important factor for older women facing osteoporosis, a condition that weakens the bones and can result in serious injury upon falling.

Cutting down on red meat helps your body detoxify, cleaning out your liver and kidneys, and controls your calorie intake, helping to maintain a healthy weight. Replacing these with fish or fibrous vegetables increases this effect. Becoming a vegetarian can have the same impact as well. Studies also recommend supplemental vitamins, especially B12 and calcium.

Having a pet is another good way to extend your life expectancy. Not only are you more likely to exercise if you're walking and playing with your pet, but those who have pets are less likely to experience depression and anxiety, both of which contribute to shorter life spans. Spending time with friends and family has a similar effect.

Quitting smoking, or avoiding it altogether, will lead to a longer life. The same applies to drinking alcohol—do so moderately or not at all to live for a long time. Drinking water, on the other hand, is very healthy and support all of the body's organs.

A few additional ways are being optimistic, doing volunteer work, and challenging your mind through stimulating activities. All of these have been shown to give someone a better outlook on life, leading to less stress, healthier habits, and stronger bodies.

Stimulating hobbies, such as reading or solving logic puzzles, has the benefit of fighting Alzheimer's disease and dementia as well as improving memory, coordination, and reducing confusion. This boosts the quality of life in old age, leading to increased longevity.

Factors that Decrease Life Expectancy

Just as there are a number of ways to ensure you live longer, there are various things that contribute to a shorter life.

Exercise, eating right, and having friends and family can increase one's life expectancy, but those who never exercise, don't eat vegetables, and spend their time alone are far more likely to die sooner.

Those who are stressed often can do a lot of damage to their bodies. Stress releases harmful hormones into the bloodstream to help you cope with the situation, but overexposure damages the heart, muscles, and brain.

Eating too much is also bad for your health. This doesn't have to be fatty foods; too much food, regardless of what it is, leads to a shorter life. Researchers found that monkeys who ate 30% less outlived the monkeys that ate more, and this was later applied to human longevity as well.

If you don't sleep enough, you're creating a compound problem. Not only does sleep increase the life span, but it lets the brain calm down from the day's activities, decreasing your overall stress level as well as feelings of depression and anxiety. Not sleeping causes you to feel more hungry more often, so your brain can get an artificial boost of energy from breaking down food, and you'll be more likely to indulge in caffeinated drinks that are loaded with fats and sugars.

Another factor here is whether or not you worry about growing older. A study suggested that those who become depressed or angry about aging lived seven years shorter than those who did not.

A less understood factor that alters life expectancy is whether or not you attend religious services. Regardless of religion, those who attend routinely live longer than those who do not.

DATA AND ANALYSES

Data

Table 32.1 Life Expectancy by Sex and Race in 2011

Average life expectancy	Hispanic	Non-Hispanic black	Non-Hispanic white	All races and origins
Male	78.9	71.6	76.4	76.3
Female	83.7	77.8	81.1	81.1
Both	81.4	74.8	78.8	78.7

Source: http://www.cdc.gov/nchs/data/databriefs/db115.htm

Analysis

Table 32.1 shows the average life expectancy, at birth, for peoples from different racial backgrounds and both sexes. It also displays the averages from these two categories. It does not consider those beneath the age of 50. In general, women live longer than men by about 5 years. However, non-Hispanic black women live six years longer than men of the same race, while white women live just 4.5 years longer. However, Hispanic people live, on average, 2.7 years longer. Men and women both live 2.6 years longer than those of the same gender. They live about six years longer than non-Hispanic black people.

Data

Table 32.2 Infant Mortality Rates From 1990 to 2010

Year	Deaths
1990	9.3
1992	8.5
1994	8.3
1996	7.4
1998	7.2
2000	7.0
2002	7.0
2004	6.9
2006	6.7
2008	6.6
2010	6.4

Source: http://www.cdc.gov/nchs/data/databriefs/db115.htm

Analysis

Table 32.2 shows the rate of infant death, measure in deaths per 1,000 live births (therefore excluding stillborn children). This is used as a measure of how healthy the population is overall, rather than focusing on specific groups such as non-Hispanic black women. Over the past two decades, the rate has dropped roughly 34%, showing that one-third as many babies are dying as before, a measure that the population's health has increased tremendously.

DISCUSSION QUESTIONS

1. There are a number of easy ways to increase life expectancy, such as taking walks or owning a pet. Which appeal most to you and why?

2. Some people consciously ignore or refuse to do some of the things that could increase one's life span, such as continuing to smoke despite knowing it could cause cancer. Why do you think someone would do this?

3. Consider the racial differences in life expectancy. What factors do you think could cause these differences?

4. Consider the gender differences in life expectancy. Why do you think women always tend to live about five years longer than men, no matter what race they are?

5. Attending religious services has a positive effect on life expectancy. What could be the reasons behind this?

33

LUNG CANCER

INTRODUCTION

Understanding Lung Cancer

The lungs provide oxygen to the body via the blood and thus play an essential role in life. When a person develops lung cancer, he or she experiences uncontrolled growth of abnormal cells in one or both or their lungs. These abnormal cells can form tumors and interfere with the proper functioning of the lungs.

There are two main types of lung cancer: non-small cell lung cancer and small cell lung cancer. These terms come from the size of the cancer cells when seen under a microscope. A small percentage of lung cancers (approximately 10–15% of all lung cancers) are small cell lung cancers. Small cell lung cancers often start in the bronchi near the center of the chest and spread rapidly throughout the body in the early stages of the disease and, as such, it is a very challenging form of cancer to treat. The vast majority of lung cancers (approximately 85–90% of all lung cancers) are non-small cell lung cancers. There are three main subtypes of non-small cell lung cancers: squamous cell carcinoma; adenocarcinoma; and large cell (undifferentiated) carcinoma. These subtypes are grouped together because their prognosis and treatment approaches are usually similar. However, the cells in these subtypes differ in chemical composition, as well as in size and shape.

Symptoms

Most people with lung cancer do not experience any significant symptoms until the cancer is advanced. When a person does experience the symptoms of lung cancer, the symptoms can often be mistaken for other, less serious ailments, such as a cold. Symptoms of lung cancer that are in the chest include:

- Coughing, especially if it persists or becomes intense
- Pain in the chest, shoulder, or back unrelated to pain from coughing
- A change in color or volume of sputum
- Shortness of breath
- Changes in the voice or being hoarse
- Harsh sounds with breathing
- Recurrent lung problems, such as bronchitis or pneumonia
- Coughing up phlegm or mucus, especially if it is tinged with blood
- Coughing up blood

Lung cancer may spread to other parts of the body, including the lymph nodes, bones, brain, liver, and adrenal glands. If the original lung cancer has spread outside of the lungs, a person may feel other symptoms, including:

- Loss of appetite or unexplained weight loss
- Cachexia (muscle wasting)
- Fatigue
- Headaches, bone, or joint pain
- Bone fractures not related to accidental injury
- Neurological symptoms, such as unsteady gait or memory loss
- Neck or facial swelling
- General weakness
- Bleeding
- Blood clots

Diagnosis

Staging lung cancer is based on whether the cancer is local or has spread from the lungs to the lymph nodes or other organs. Because the lungs are large, tumors can grow in them for a long time before they are found. Even when symptoms do occur, people often think they are due to other causes. For this reason, early-stage lung cancer is usually difficult to detect. Most people with lung cancer are diagnosed at stages III and IV. By this time, the disease has typically progressed to such an extent that treatment becomes very challenging.

As with all cancers, lung cancer survival rates can be improved with early testing and screening. With respect to lung cancer, researchers are examining three main tests to determine their usefulness in decreasing the risks of dying from lung cancer: chest x-ray; sputum cytology; low-dose spiral CT scan. A chest X-ray is an X-ray of the organs and bones inside the chest. Sputum cytology is a procedure in which a sample of sputum (mucus that is coughed up from the lungs) is viewed under a microscope to check for cancer cells. Low-dose spiral CT scan, also called a low-dose helical CT scan, is a procedure that uses low-dose radiation to make a series of very detailed pictures of areas inside the body. It uses an X-ray machine that scans the body in a spiral path. Current research suggests that of these three tests, only screening with low-dose spiral CT scans has been shown to decrease the risk of dying from lung cancer.

If, as a result of a screening procedure, lung cancer is suspected, a biopsy is performed on a small piece of tissue from the lung. By reviewing the cells under a microscope, the physician is able to determine whether the cells are cancerous and is also able to determine the type of cancer involved.

Risk Factors

Smoking is widely recognized as the leading cause of lung cancer but there are other risk factors as well. The primary risk factors for the development of lung cancer are:

- Smoking cigarettes, pipes, or cigars (currently or in the past)
- Being exposed to secondhand smoke
- Having a family history of lung cancer
- Being treated with radiation therapy to the breast or chest
- Being exposed to asbestos, chromium, nickel, arsenic, soot, or tar
- Being exposed to radon in the home
- Living where there is air pollution.
- Being HIV positive
- Using beta carotene supplements and being a heavy smoker

Treatment

Individuals afflicted with non-small cell lung cancer may be treated with surgery, radiation, chemotherapy, and targeted treatments, either alone or in combination. Each of these types of treatments may cause different side effects. For people with small cell lung cancer, regardless of stage, chemotherapy is the primary form of treatment. Radiation treatment may be used as well depending on the stage of cancer.

DATA AND ANALYSES

Data

Table 33.1 Incidence of Lung Cancer Compared With Other Types of Cancers

Common types of cancer	Estimated new cases 2013	Estimated deaths 2013
Prostate cancer	238,590	29,720
Breast cancer	232,340	39,620
Lung and bronchus cancer	228,190	159,480
Colon and rectum cancer	142,820	50,830
Melanoma of the skin	76,690	9,480
Bladder cancer	72,570	15,210
Non-Hodgkin lymphoma	69,740	19,020
Kidney and renal pelvis cancer	65,150	13,680
Thyroid cancer	60,220	1,850
Endometrial cancer	49,560	8,190

Source: http://seer.cancer.gov/statfacts/html/lungb.html

Analysis

Lung cancer is a fairly common type of cancer. It is the third most common type of cancer, following prostate and breast cancer. At present, lung and bronchus cancer represents 13.7% of all new cancer cases in the United States. Unfortunately, it is also the most deadly cancer.

Data

Table 33.2 Tracking Number of New Cases and Deaths per 100,000 People (all races, males and females), Age-adjusted

Year	New cases—SEER 9	New cases—SEER 13	Deaths—U.S.
1975	52.3	—	42.6
1976	55.4	—	44.2
1977	56.7	—	45.5
1978	57.8	—	46.9
1979	58.6	—	47.7
1980	60.7	—	49.4
1981	62.0	—	50.0
1982	63.3	—	51.4
1983	63.5	—	52.4
1984	65.5	—	53.4
1985	64.6	—	54.3
1986	65.8	—	55.0
1987	67.9	—	56.2
1988	68.0	—	57.0
1989	67.5	—	57.9
1990	68.1	—	58.9
1991	69.2	—	59.0
1992	69.4	67.0	58.9
1993	67.8	65.7	59.1
1994	67.2	64.7	58.5
1995	66.8	64.9	58.4
1996	66.5	64.4	57.9
1997	66.6	63.8	57.5
1998	67.5	64.4	57.1
1999	65.8	62.9	55.4
2000	64.1	60.8	55.8
2001	64.1	60.8	55.3
2002	64.0	60.3	55.0
2003	64.7	60.6	54.2
2004	62.2	58.6	53.4
2005	63.0	59.0	52.9
2006	62.2	57.9	51.7
2007	61.9	57.5	50.7
2008	60.2	55.9	49.6
2009	59.5	55.6	48.4
2010	56.7	52.4	47.4

Source: http://seer.cancer.gov/statfacts/html/ld/lungb.html

Analysis

Table 33.2 makes reference to SEER 9 and SEER 13. Before analyz-
ing the substance of the data presented in the above chart, a brief
explanation of SEER data is required. The Surveillance, Epidemiology, and End Results (SEER) Program of the National Cancer Institute provides detailed information on cancer statistics. SEER began
collecting data on cancer cases on January 1, 1973, in the states of
Connecticut, Iowa, New Mexico, Utah, and Hawaii and the metropolitan areas of Detroit and San Francisco-Oakland and continued
to expand from there. The SEER 9 registries are Atlanta, Connecticut, Detroit, Hawaii, Iowa, New Mexico, San Francisco-Oakland,
Seattle-Puget Sound, and Utah. The SEER 11 registries consist of the
SEER 9, as described above, plus Los Angeles and San Jose-Monterey.
The SEER 13 registries consist of the SEER 11, as described above,
plus rural Georgia and the Alaska Native Tumor Registry.

By reviewing the number of new cases of lung cancer and the
number of deaths from lung cancer, we can analyze statistics over
time and see whether progress is made in reducing the lung cancer rates and the number of deaths from lung cancer. Data shows
that between 2000 and 2010 in the regions covered by the identified
registries, rates for new lung and bronchus cancer cases have been
falling on average 1.3% each year and deaths from lung cancer have
been falling on average 1.7% during this ten-year period.

When studying diseases such as lung cancer, it can be very useful
to track the number of new cases and deaths over time. This information can help researchers and public health workers to determine where progress is and is not being made and to determine
whether additional research and/or interventions are needed to
address various challenges.

Data

Table 33.3 Lung and Bronchus Cancer Incidence Rates* by State, 2010

Incidence rates	States
26.8 to 56.9	Arizona, California, Colorado, Hawaii, Idaho, Montana, New Jersey, New Mexico, North Dakota, Oregon, Texas, Utah, and Wyoming
57.0 to 63.2	Connecticut, District of Columbia, Florida, Kansas, Maryland, Nebraska, Nevada, New York, South Dakota, Virginia, Washington, and Wisconsin

Incidence rates	States
63.3 to 68.4	Alaska, Delaware, Georgia, Illinois, Iowa, Massachusetts, New Hampshire, Ohio, Oklahoma, Pennsylvania, Rhode Island, and South Carolina
68.5 to 97.3	Alabama, Indiana, Kentucky, Louisiana, Maine, Michigan, Mississippi, Missouri, North Carolina, Tennessee, Vermont, and West Virginia
Data not available[‡]	Arkansas and Minnesota

[*] Rates are per 100,000 and are age-adjusted to the 2000 U.S. standard population.
[‡] Rates are not shown if the state did not meet USCS publication criteria or if the state did not submit data to CDC.

Source: http://www.cdc.gov/cancer/lung/statistics/state.htm

Analysis

In the United States, lung cancer rates vary from state to state. As Table 33.3 indicates, rates of lung cancer tend to be lower in the western portion of the United States, with the highest rates occurring in states located in the South and near the center of the country.

DISCUSSION QUESTIONS

1. Lung cancer is the leading cause of cancer death in the United States. What are some possible reasons for this?
2. Table 33.2 shows that rates for new lung cancer cases and death rates have both been falling. What are some possible reasons for the decline in lung cancer rates and deaths from lung cancer?
3. Some, but not all cases of lung cancer are caused by behavioral factors, including the use of tobacco. Do you believe that our public health system has done enough to make people aware of the risks of tobacco use? If not, what else can and should be done?
4. One challenge of lung cancer treatment is that by the time the cancer is discovered, the disease has often progressed to such a point that effective treatment becomes very difficult. How can our health system improve lung cancer screening?
5. Lung cancer afflicts more men than women. What are some possible reasons for the gender differences in lung cancer?

34

MAMMOGRAMS

INTRODUCTION

Understanding Mammograms

There are several different screening tests, or methods of detecting or locating, cancer that range from blood tests to tissue analysis, among many others. For some cancers, there are specific screening tests that can be very effective in reducing mortality from the cancer. One such test is the mammogram, which is used primarily to detect breast cancer. There are also diagnostic mammograms, which are more detailed screening tests that are meant to diagnose breast cancer. It is worth mentioning that mammography, along with breast cancer, is usually associated with women. However, on far less frequent occasions, men can also decide to be screened or diagnosed via mammogram if a doctor suspects they are at risk for breast cancer.

A mammogram is an example of an imaging screening test, which, as its name suggests, involves the use of an X-ray machine to generate a picture. This is done by putting the breast on a plastic plate, applying pressure and flattening it with another plate from above, and projecting X-rays onto it. The radiologist administering the mammogram will take at least four pictures of each breast to check for any kind of early signs of breast cancer and will usually be able to release the results within weeks.

Mammograms have been found to detect the early signs of breast cancer years before they become noticeable to the person or too unbearable for them to participate in normal daily activities. This method of screening for cancer is helpful because it has the potential to save lives, allowing a woman to obtain the proper treatment to remove the breast cancer cells in her body before they spread to other areas.

Guidelines

Many of the guidelines given to women who are considering or have planned to get a mammogram are directly related to statistics on breast cancer. For example, because breast cancer is widely known to affect women with a family history of breast cancer, as well as older women, doctors recommend scheduling a mammogram every two years for women over 50 years old. This usually ensures that lumps or other suspicious areas that appear in the breasts with age are not cancerous. Cancer experts usually recommend women over 74 years old to discontinue routine screening via mammography. Although it is possible for women over the age of 74 years to contract breast cancer, it is outside the most at-risk age range. Perhaps most importantly, a facility must be approved by the U.S. Food and Drug Administration to perform mammograms.

Variables

No two mammograms are alike. There are many variables that make each X-ray image taken during the screening test different. These variables, whether or not they can be changed or controlled, have the potential to influence the breast image and even the result of the mammogram test. The main variables involved in mammograms include:

- Patient characteristics, including age and breast density
- Tumor characteristics, including the appearance of breast cancer cells as normal breast tissue
- Radiologist characteristics, including level of expertise
- Facility characteristics, including screening protocol

Risks and Effects

A screening test like a mammogram may seem harmless, especially since it is considered an effective preventative measure against breast cancer mortality. However, there are actually certain risks associated with getting one. According to the National Cancer Institute, the most common risks and effects of mammography use include:

- Discomfort
- Overdiagnosis
- Radiation exposure
- Anxiety
- False-positive results
- Additional intervention brought on by false-positive results
- False-negative results
- False sense of security related to false-negative results

DATA AND ANALYSES

Data

Table 34.1 Percentage of U.S. Women Aged 50–74 Years Who Reported Having a Mammogram by Race and Ethnicity, 2010

Race or ethnicity	Percentage
Black	73.2
White	72.8
American Indian/Alaska Native	69.4
Asian	64.1
Non-Hispanic	72.7
Hispanic	69.7

Note: Data takes into account mammograms that were done within two years of the survey being taken.

Source: http://www.cdc.gov/cancer/breast/statistics/screening.htm

Analysis

Table 34.1 shows the percentage of U.S. women of different races and ethnicities and between the ages of 50 and 74 who reported having a mammogram within two years. It is worth noting that women in the 50–74 age group are more at risk for breast cancer, especially certain invasive types, than younger women.

In general, all of the races and ethnicities fell in the 60–70% range. This shows that a majority of women in this age group, regardless of their race or ethnicity, decide to use mammography as a method of breast cancer screening. Although all race and ethnicity groups were very close in percentage, some were, of course, higher than others. While Asian women made up the group with the lowest percentage of 64.1%, black women made up the group with the highest percentage of 73.2%.

Data

Table 34.2 Percentage of U.S. Women Who Reported Mammography Use, Selected Years Between 1987 and 2010

Year	40 to 49 years	50 to 64 years	65 years and older
1987	31.9	31.7	22.8
1990	55.1	56.0	43.4
1993	59.9	65.1	54.2
1994	61.3	66.5	55.0
2000	64.3	78.7	67.9
2003	64.4	76.2	67.7
2005	63.5	71.8	63.8
2008	61.5	74.2	65.5
2010	62.3	72.6	64.4

Source: http://www.cdc.gov/nchs/data/hus/2013/083.pdf

Analysis

Table 34.2 shows a timeline of selected years between 1987 and 2010, and the percentage of United States women in three age groups (40–49 years, 50–64 years, and ≥65 years) who reported using mammography as a breast cancer screening method during those years.

With each consecutive year recorded, all three age groups surveyed showed an increase of women using mammography. In fact, comparing percentages in 1987 and 2010, the numbers doubled for the 50–64 year age range (31.7% in 1987 and 72.6% in 2010) and tripled in the ≥65 year age group (22.8% in 1987 and 64.4% in 2010).

Data

Table 34.3 Number of Screening Mammography Examinations With Corresponding Cancer Rate and Cancer Detection Rate by Months Since Previous Mammography, From 2004 to 2008

Race or ethnicity	Number of screening mammography examinations	Cancer rate	Cancer detection rate
Total	1,838,372	4.91	4.14
9–15 months	1,001,975	4.26	3.41
16–20 months	238,829	4.62	3.93
21–27 months	250,569	5.50	4.86
28+ months	266,856	6.50	6.23
No previous mammography	80,143	5.37	4.77

Note: Data in table for both cancer rate and cancer detection rate is calculated per 1,000 examinations.

Source: Breast Cancer Surveillance Consortium (HHSN261201100031C). http://breastscreening.cancer.gov

Analysis

Table 34.3 references 1,838,372 mammograms administered during the four year time frame from 2004 to 2008. This data is accompanied by the breast cancer rate—the number of cancers among the examinations—as well as the breast cancer detection rate—the number of cancers with a positive initial interpretation—corresponding with the amount of time since the woman's last mammogram.

The data shows no significant trend, although the cancer rates and cancer detection rates are all in the 3.4–6.5 range. The cancer rate is always shown to be larger than the cancer detection rate, albeit a small apparent difference between the numbers.

DISCUSSION QUESTIONS

1. Mammography utilizes a low dose of radiation that is minimally harmful when it comes in contact with most women's bodies. How would the effects of a mammogram on a woman's body be different if it required a high dose of radiation?
2. Mammograms are screening tests that are key in detecting breast cancer early. What other kinds of screening tests for cancer are you familiar with?

3. According to Table 34.2, the percentage of women in the United States who reported having a recent mammogram steadily increased over the course of more than two decades. What are some possible reasons for the fact that more women decided to have a mammogram in 2010 than in 1987?

4. Women who are scheduling a mammogram are usually advised by doctors not to come in the week before or the week of the start of their menstruation cycles. Using what you know about related changes in a woman's body, why might doing a mammogram during this time not be ideal?

5. Some medical professionals question the utility of mammography and consider it an unreliable method of detecting breast cancer. What method of cancer screening might doctors who discredit mammography recommend instead?

35

MENTAL HEALTH

INTRODUCTION

Mental health is a term that generally describes whether your brain is able to think through things and control your moods correctly. Stress and anxiety levels, mood stability, impulse control, substance use or disuse, and your senses can all be factors in assessing mental health.

Someone with good mental health tends to be happier, able to process emotions well, and can deal with stress in a normal manner. If they smoke or drink, they do so in moderation, and they don't use illicit drugs like heroin or cocaine. They also obey laws and do not look to hurt others.

A person with poor mental health may be bitter, angry, depressed, violent, or suicidal. They may take out stress through being verbally or physically abusive toward others, or they may internalize it and harm themselves. Such people may have panic attacks, smoke or drink excessively, or use illegal drugs. Law breaking behavior is common as well. Those who make a pattern of such behavior often suffer from a mental illness.

It is important to note that it can be hard to tell the symptoms of poor mental health from the actual diagnosis. For instance, people suffering from depression may drink too much alcohol, but people who drink too much alcohol may then suffer from depression while drunk or while suffering from withdrawal.

How to Maintain Good Mental Health

In order to ensure you stay healthy, stress free, and have low mental illness risk factors, you can do a wide variety of things that will improve your overall well-being.

The best way is to be social. Having strong connections to friends and family reduces stress and elevates your mood. It also gives you an opportunity to talk about issues that are bothering you, removing additional stress. They may even be able to solve your problems. In return, caring for others has also been shown to increase a person's sense of accomplishment, so sometimes helping others helps you too.

Doing volunteer work, as well as pursuing hobbies, have also been shown to improve a person's mental health. Doing one of these provides a sense of skill and purpose. Having a strong network of friends adds to this effect because they can then comment on how positive or talented you are, providing an external as well as internal reward. If you challenge yourself to a new goal or learning a new skill, meeting this challenge will not only cause you to feel proud of yourself, you will have something new and impressive to talk about.

Eating right, getting enough rest, and exercising are also key components of a healthy mind. By ensuring your body is free of toxins and full of nutrients, you make sure your brain can process emotions correctly, reducing the likelihood of stress and mental illness.

Types of Mental Illness

There are several types of mental illnesses, the most common being anxiety disorders, mood disorders, psychotic disorders, eating disorders, and impulse control, and addiction disorders.

Anxiety disorders feature a degree of inappropriate fear in various situations. Some people might feel afraid all the time (general anxiety disorder), be very afraid of certain things like puppies or blue cars (specific phobia), or feel anxiety that is only calmed by ritualistic behavior (obsessive compulsive disorder). These are often accompanied by physical symptoms like sweating, a rapid heart rate, or shaking.

Mood disorders pertain to persistent sadness (depression) or periods of being overly happy (mania), as well as a fluctuation between the two. The most well-known of these is bipolar disorder.

Psychotic disorders involve an altered perception of reality or abnormal thought pattern. Those who suffer from these typically experience hallucinations—when they see, hear or otherwise experience something that is not real—and delusions—a belief in something extraordinary or impossible despite evidence that proves the belief is false. Schizophrenia is the most common example of this.

Eating disorders focus on severe and debilitating attitudes regarding weight and food. The most common of these are anorexia nervosa, most commonly identified by starving one's self to lose weight, and bulimia nervosa, most often associated with throwing up after eating.

Impulse control disorders are indicated by the inability to resist the urge to do things that could hurt others, and are often known by names with 'mania' at the end. Pyromania, an obsession with starting fires, and kleptomania, the uncontrollable impulse to steal, are two very common impulse disorders.

Symptoms of Mental Health Disorders

There are a number of general symptoms that can indicate an underlying mental disorder. Some of these include:

- Confused thinking
- Periods of inexplicable sadness
- Irritability
- Excessive worry
- Social withdrawal
- Intense anger
- Suicidal thoughts
- Unexplained physical illness
- Inability to cope with daily problems
- Delusions or hallucinations
- Dramatic changes to sleeping or eating habits
- Abuse of drugs or alcohol

DATA AND ANALYSES

Data

Table 35.1 Average Age at First Use Among Alcohol and Illicit Drug Use Initiates Ages 12 to 49

	Alcohol	Illicit drugs
2007	16.8	18.0
2008	17.0	18.8

(Continued)

Table 35.1 Average Age at First Use among Alcohol and Illicit Drug Use Initiates Ages 12 to 49 (*Continued*)

	Alcohol	Illicit drugs
2009	16.9	17.6
2010	17.1	19.1
2011	17.1	18.1

Source: http://www.samhsa.gov/data/2012BehavioralHealthUS/2012-BHUS.pdf

Analysis

Table 35.1 shows an interesting difference between alcohol and drug use. While alcohol was commonly used at almost the same age by all those who responded, drug use varied significantly. The range of alcohol use was only 0.3 years while the range for illicit drugs was 1.5 years, indicating a very wide scope for when people begin to use such drugs.

A person's first use of alcohol appears to occur during or just before one's senior year of high school, while drug use appears toward the end or during one's first year in college.

Data

Table 35.2 Lifetime Prevalence of Selected Mental Health Disorder Classes Among Adults, by Age Group, by Percent

	Age 18–29	Age 30–44	Age 45–59	Age 60 or older
Mood disorders	21.4	24.6	22.9	11.9
Anxiety disorders	30.2	35.1	30.8	15.3
Impulse control disorders	26.8	23.0	Not given	Not given

Source: http://www.samhsa.gov/data/2012BehavioralHealthUS/2012-BHUS.pdf

Analysis

Table 35.2 shows the incidence of mental health disorders among all persons over the age of 18, meaning this group is subjected to the natural and social stressors accompanying adulthood.

While mood disorders appeared fairly consistently over the human lifespan, only half of the population of this group demonstrated the previous ranges' occurrence of about 22–23%. Due to the severity of mood disorders and the mortality rate that accompanies them, this may be due to such persons passing away before reaching this age.

Anxiety disorders spike between ages 30 and 44, the years during which an adult is most likely to be competing for a good job and raising children. However, not enough information is presented about the population of the study to determine what the cause of this spike may actually be. The notable drop in anxiety disorders among the 60+ population can indicate that these disorders are reduced in prevalence and severity as social pressures are reduced.

Impulse control disorders are shown dropping from the 18–29 age range into the 30–44 age range, suggesting that overcoming them may be a matter of learning to deal with them, but because the occurrence of these was not tracked above the age of 45, this trend cannot be confirmed.

Data

Table 35.3 Lifetime Prevalence of Selected Mental Health Disorder Classes Among Adolescents, by Age Group, by Percent

	Age 13–14	Age 15–16	Age 17–18
Mood disorders	10.5	15.5	18.1
Anxiety disorders	31.4	32.1	32.3
Impulse control disorders	18.2	19.5	21.9

Source: http://www.samhsa.gov/data/2012BehavioralHealthUS/2012-BHUS.pdf

Analysis

Table 35.3 tracks the incidence of the three major mental disorder groups among the adolescent population. All three groups are shown increasing as the subject grew older, with mood disorders increasing the most and anxiety increasing the least. One is most susceptible to developing a mental disorder, especially a mood disorder, between ages 13 and 18, so the fact that mood disorders increase so drastically is to be expected.

However, anxiety disorders had the highest rate of prevalence while mood disorders had the lowest, suggesting that persons at these ages are generally quite anxious, possibly about grades, entering college, leaving home, and a variety of other social pressures.

DISCUSSION QUESTIONS

1. Alcohol, cigarettes. and drug use can trigger mental illness, but can also be symptoms of mental illness. Do you believe enough is done to educate people on this connection?

2. Being close to friends and family reduces the incidence of mental illness, but many mentally ill people have these connections. Why do you think this helps some but not others?

3. A person's first experience with alcohol tends to be at age 17—roughly the same age at which adolescent mood disorders become the most prevalent, which can be dangerous if that person later depends on alcohol to cope with mood swings. What can be done to educate young people about this connection?

4. Anxiety disorders peak among 30–44-year-olds. How can we reduce work and family stress, or make sure these people cope effectively enough to lower the incidence of anxiety disorders?

5. People who suffer from mental illness can be tough for others to be around, especially if that person is very controlling, anxious or angry. What can be done to help those who drive away the friends or family that might support them?

36

OBESITY

INTRODUCTION

Understanding Obesity

Body weight consists of weight from muscle, bone, fat, and body water. The terms *obesity* and *overweight* both indicate that an individual's weight is higher than the recommended healthy weight for their height; however, the terms differ. Being overweight means that an individual weighs too much. Being obese means that an individual weighs too much specifically because of excess body fat.

Healthy recommended body weights can be calculated using the body mass index (BMI). BMIs are calculated by dividing an individual's weight in kilograms by their height in meters squared. Obesity is categorized as presenting a BMI of 30 or greater. However, BMI does not directly measure body fat, so some exceptions may be athletes that consist mainly of muscle.

Obesity occurs over time as more calories are eaten than burned. Obesity is a serious condition, as it increases the risk of many other health problems, such as heart disease, diabetes, arthritis, and high blood pressure. However, losing just 5–10% of an obese body weight can prevent health complications.

Symptoms

Many people first notice that they have gained weight when they no longer fit in their clothes, they recognized extra body fat around their waist, or the number on the scale increases. Besides presenting a BMI of 30 or greater, there are not many other symptoms of obesity; however, many health complications can arise from being obese. Symptoms of developed health complications may be noticed and should be addressed if an individual is obese.

Risk Factors

Typically, obesity occurs due to a variety of factors. Obesity can be influenced by genetics and hormonal factors, as genes affect the amount of body fat that one stores and where it is distributed, as well as how efficiently the body converts food into energy and burns calories while exercising. However, the main causes of obesity are controllable lifestyle factors, such as diet and exercise.

Unhealthy diet and eating habits contributes to weight gain, as the body stores excess calories as fat. Inactivity also leads to weight gain, as less calories are burned than consumed. Lack of sleep can also alter hormones, increasing an individual's appetite and craving for foods that are high in calories and carbohydrates. Family lifestyles are important as well, as eating and exercise habits are often mimicked within families. Also, though obesity can occur at any age, the risk becomes higher as individuals age, for their hormones change and they may become less active, with lower muscle mass. Socioeconomic factors may also lead to weight gain, as people may not be educated on healthy diet habits or have the money to purchase healthier foods. Additional contributors to weight gain include quitting smoking, pregnancy, and certain medications if they are not complimented with a healthy diet or exercise. Such medications include certain antidepressants, diabetes medications, antiseizure medications, antipsychotic medications, corticosteroids, and beta blockers.

Diagnosis

Certain tests will be performed if an individual's BMI is in the overweight or obese range to check for any complications that can arise due to obesity. An individual's BMI should be calculated at least once a year. Typically, a general physical exam will be performed to measure height; check vital signs such as heart rate, blood pressure, and temperature; listen to the heart and lungs; and examine the abdomen. The history of an individual's health may also be examined, including weight history, exercise habits, eating habits, medications, stress levels, family history, and other present conditions. To check for additional present conditions, such as high blood pressure or diabetes, laboratory tests may be ordered. Such tests may include a cholesterol test, liver function test, fasting glucose test, thyroid test, or heart test. Certain examinations, such as measuring waist circumference, may also indicate additional conditions such as diabetes or heart disease.

Treatment

The goal of treating obesity is to reach and maintain a healthy weight. A team of medical professionals can help identify and maintain healthy eating and exercise habits. Typically, the first goal is to lose 3–5% of total body weight. Specific treatment methods depend on an individual's BMI and overall health, as well as their commitment to a healthy diet and exercise plan. The main methods that are used to treat obesity include dietary changes, increased exercise, behavioral changes, prescription weight-loss medications, and weight-loss surgeries. Slow and steady weight loss is the best way to reach and maintain a healthy weight, as crash dieting or fad diets can often lead to a reoccurrence of weight gain.

Reducing calories and substituting healthy foods are a key component of treating obesity. To reduce calories, an individual can start by logging a typical day's consumption of food and drink. Determining when and what an individual consumes will help them reasonably cut back. Typically, females who are trying to lose weight should consume 1,200–1,500 calories per day, while males who are trying to lose weight should consume 1,500–1,800 calories per day. Educating oneself about healthy nutrition will also help determine what foods should be consumed to aid weight loss, such as vegetables and lean sources of protein.

Physical exercise will also help reach and maintain a weight-loss goal. It is recommended to get at least 150 minutes a week of exercise at a moderate intensity; however, individuals who are serious about losing weight may need to exercise for 300 or more minutes per week. When beginning physical activity, certain methods such as breaking up exercises throughout the day or exercising with a partner may help individuals keep their commitment. Though aerobic exercise is the most efficient for weight loss, even daily changes can help lose weight, such as parking further away from a destination or choosing the stairs over the elevator.

Behavioral changes can occur after determining what factors contribute to an individual's obesity, such as stress, living situations, or lack of time to exercise. Counseling and therapy may be needed to address emotional issues related to food consumption and to maintain behavioral changes. Ways to cope may also be offered through therapy. There are many options for individuals who seek counseling for obesity, such as support groups.

Prescription weight-loss medications may be recommended if an individual is not seeing progress after the development of healthy lifestyle changes and if their BMI is greater than 30. Individuals who have a BMI of 27 or greater may also be recommended to a prescription if their obesity has caused other health problems, such as diabetes or high blood pressure. Prescription weight-loss medications need to be closely monitored and accompanied by consistent physical exercise and a healthy diet.

Weight-loss surgery, also known as bariatric surgery, is another alternative to treating obesity. Weight-loss surgeries limit the amount of food that an individual is able to eat or decreases the absorption of calories. Surgery may be recommended if an individual has a BMI of 40 or greater, or if their BMI is 35–39.9 and has caused additional health problems. Individuals who undergo weight-loss surgery must be committed maintaining a healthy diet and exercise even after the surgery. Options for weight-loss surgery include gastric bypass surgery, which creates small pouch at top of stomach that is connected directly to the small intestine; laparoscopic adjustable gastric banding, which separates the stomach in two pouches with inflatable band; gastric sleeve, which removes a large portion of the stomach; and biliopancreatic diversion with duodenal switch, which also removes a large portion of the stomach. All weight-loss surgeries have risks that should be discussed with a medical professional.

DATA AND ANALYSES

Data

Table 36.1 Obesity Prevalence by Age and Gender: United States, 2009–2010

Age	Prevalence in males (%)	Prevalence in females (%)	Total prevalence (%)
2–5 years	14.4	9.6	12.1
6–11 years	20.1	15.7	18.0
12–19 years	19.6	17.1	18.4

Age	Prevalence in males (%)	Prevalence in females (%)	Total prevalence (%)
20–39 years	33.2	31.9	32.6
40–59 years	37.2	36.0	36.6
60 years and older	36.6	42.3	39.7

Source: Carroll, M.D., Flegal, K.M., Kit, B.K., & Ogden, C.L. 2012. "Prevalence of obesity in the United States, 2009–2010." Centers for Disease Control and Prevention. Retrieved from: http://www.cdc.gov/nchs/data/databriefs/db82.htm

Analysis

Almost 41 million females and over 37 million males ages 20 and older were obese between 2009 and 2010. Additionally, among individuals aged 2–19 years old, over five million females and nearly seven million males were obese. Though there was no change in the prevalence of obesity between 2007–2008 and 2009–2010, these statistics represent approximately one-third of adults and almost 17% of children.

In general, when broken down by gender, there is not a great difference between prevalence of obesity in females and males. By age, it is apparent that obesity prevalence increases as individuals get older. Almost 40% of individuals aged 60 and older were obese in 2009–2010. Among males, there was no significant difference in obesity prevalence by age; however, females aged 60 and older presented a prevalence of 42.3%, which was much higher than younger females. Additionally, adolescents above the age of six presented a significantly higher obesity prevalence than children under the age of six.

Data

Table 36.2 Obesity Prevalence by Race/ethnicity and Gender: United States, 2011–2012

Race/ethnicity	Prevalence in males (%)	Prevalence in females (%)	Total prevalence (%)
Non-Hispanic white	32.4	32.8	32.6
Non-Hispanic black	37.1	56.6	47.8
Non-Hispanic Asian	10.0	11.4	10.8
Hispanic	40.1	44.4	42.5

Source: Carroll, M.D., Flegal, K.M., Kit, B.K., & Ogden, C.L. 2013. "Prevalence of obesity among adults: United States, 2011–2012." Centers for Disease Control and Prevention. Retrieved from: http://www.cdc.gov/nchs/data/databriefs/db131.htm

Analysis

Table 36.2 presents the prevalence of obesity between 2011 and 2012 broken down by race/ethnicity and gender. The data shows that there was not a significant difference in the prevalence of obesity between females and males, though females were slightly higher. However, Non-Hispanic black females did present a significant increase in obesity prevalence at nearly 60%, while only about 37% of Non-Hispanic black males presented obesity. In total, obesity prevalence was highest among Non-Hispanic black individuals, followed by Hispanics, Non-Hispanic whites, and Non-Hispanic Asians. Non-Hispanic Asians presented a significantly lower obesity prevalence, at only about 11%. This publication indicated that national obesity prevalence estimates for Non-Hispanic Asians were possible for the first time with this data, which may have an impact on the low rates. Further research can examine genetic factors that may describe why Non-Hispanic Asians present such a low prevalence of obesity.

DISCUSSION QUESTIONS

1. Why does obesity prevalence increase with age? How can obesity levels be decreased and maintained in older age?
2. Does the high prevalence of obesity in older adults have an impact on obesity prevalence in younger individuals? How can more healthy eating and exercise habits be implemented from a young age?
3. Why do Non-Hispanic Asian individuals present the lowest obesity prevalence? What factors contribute to their lower comparative weight?
4. Why do Non-Hispanic black females present such a high prevalence of obesity? How can this rate be decreased?
5. Why do females present a slightly higher prevalence of obesity than males?

37

PANCREATIC CANCER

INTRODUCTION

Understanding Pancreatic Cancer

The pancreas is a glandular organ associated with the digestive and endocrine systems of the human body. Located in the abdomen behind the stomach, its three sections—the head, body, and tail—work together to digest consumed food and produce hormones like glucagon and insulin to help regulate blood sugar levels. When the tissues of the pancreas are attacked by malignant cancer cells, this important organ's ability to fulfill these tasks becomes hindered or completely compromised.

There are different types of pancreatic cancer, which include glucagonoma, insulinoma, VIPoma, and islet cell tumors. These all deal with different changes in hormone production and can either be malignant or benign. For example, the very rare glucagonoma tumor produces excess glucagon in the blood, insulinoma tumors produce too much insulin, and VIPoma tumors produce surplus vasoactive intestinal peptide hormones in the intestines.

Symptoms

Pancreatic cancer is not easily detected or distinguished. Tumors in the pancreas cause symptoms that noticeable mainly during advanced stages. As is the case with many other types of cancer, including lung cancer, any significant symptoms that do appear in the early stages of pancreatic cancer might easily be mistaken for other, less serious ailments and are oftentimes ignored. Moreover, the pancreas is located in an inconvenient spot behind other organs, which make it difficult to examine. General symptoms of pancreatic cancer include but are not limited to:

- Jaundice
- Clay-colored stool
- Dark urine
- Pain in the abdomen or back
- Inexplicable weight loss
- Loss of appetite
- Diarrhea
- Increase in blood sugar
- Fatigue

In addition to these general symptoms, there are several others that are exclusive to the specific type of pancreatic cancer a person has. For example, glucagonoma patients might exhibit sudden intolerance to glucose, crusty or scaly skin rashes or lesions, excessive thirst, and inflamed mouth or tongue. Insulinoma patients, on the other hand, might exhibit behavioral changes, clouded vision, convulsions, and rapid heart rate. Finally, while islet cell tumor patients tend to shake and sweat, VIPoma patients may experience abdominal pain, flushing of the face, and nausea.

Diagnosis

There are several methods that can help doctors find a pancreatic tumor. Among these, imaging tests like CT scans, MRIs, and ultrasounds are the most common. Blood tests can also be conducted to check elevated levels of tumor markers.

Because these methods do not always provide a definitive diagnosis, a biopsy is usually performed to accurately identify pancreatic tumors. During biopsy procedures, a small section of the tumor is removed, and its cells are examined under a microscope. A biopsy is the crucial first step before further treatment is arranged.

Risk Factors

Although the exact cause of pancreatic cancer is unknown, there are several risk factors that scientists have pinpointed to identify people who are more susceptible to contracting the cancer. The risk factors associated with pancreatic cancer include:

- Smoking cigarettes
- Being obese
- Being overweight
- Having diabetes
- Having chronic pancreatitis
- Maintaining a diet high in fat
- Having a family history of pancreatic cancer
- Being exposed to certain chemicals over a long period of time

Treatment

Treatment options for patients suffering with pancreatic cancer depend on a variety of factors, including the size of the tumor, whether or not it has spread, if it has recurred or shown up for the first time, and whether the patient is physically and mentally able to undergo surgery.

Generally, the best way to ensure that the pancreatic cancer will not come back is through surgery, which completely removes the tumor from the pancreas before it spreads to other parts of the body. Unfortunately, patients whose pancreatic tumors have spread aggressively must rely on palliative treatments instead of surgery to reduce or delay symptoms that cause them pain. Introducing endoscopic plastic or metal stents, which are mesh tubes that help relieve blocked bile ducts caused by the pancreatic tumor, is a very common palliative procedure for inoperable patients.

DATA AND ANALYSES

Data

Table 37.1 Estimated New Cases and Deaths for Several Types of Cancer in the United States, 2013

Common types of cancer	Estimated new cases 2013	Estimated deaths 2013
Prostate cancer	238,590	29,720
Breast cancer	232,340	39,620
Lung and bronchus cancer	228,190	159,480
Colon and rectum cancer	142,820	50,830
Melanoma of the skin	76,690	9,480

(Continued)

Table 37.1 Estimated New Cases and Deaths for Several Types of Cancer in the United States, 2013 (*Continued*)

Common types of cancer	Estimated new cases 2013	Estimated deaths 2013
Bladder cancer	72,570	15,210
Non-Hodgkin lymphoma	69,740	19,020
Kidney and renal pelvis cancer	65,150	13,680
Thyroid cancer	60,220	1,850
Endometrial cancer	49,560	8,190
Leukemia	48,610	23,720
Pancreatic cancer	**45,220**	**38,460**

Source: http://seer.cancer.gov/statfacts/html/pancreas.html

Analysis

Pancreatic cancer is a relatively rare cancer. Table 37.1 indicates that there were 45,220 new cases of pancreatic cancer estimated in 2013. This leaves it out of the top ten common types of cancer and accounts for a 193,370 difference when compared to prostate cancer, which tops the list with 238,590 estimated new cases.

Although pancreatic cancer did rank twelfth in number of estimated new cases compared to other cancer types in 2013, it actually ranked fourth in estimated deaths that same year, with approximately 38,460 deaths that placed it after 159,480 estimated lung and bronchus cancer deaths, 50,830 estimated colon and rectum cancer deaths, and 39,620 estimated breast cancer deaths. This supports the fact that pancreatic cancer continues to be the fourth leading cause of cancer deaths in the United States.

Data

Table 37.2 Five-year Relative Survival Rate of Pancreatic Cancer Patients, Selected Years from 1975 to 2005

Year	5-year relative survival rate
1975	3.0%
1980	3.3%
1985	3.2%
1989	3.3%
1993	3.5%
1997	5.0%
2001	5.0%
2005	6.1%

Source: http://seer.cancer.gov/statfacts/html/pancreas.html

Analysis

Table 37.2 tracks the changes in the five-year relative survival rate of people who have been diagnosed with pancreatic cancer in the United States during selected years between 1975 and 2005. Overall, the five-year relative survival rate has increased from 3.0% in 1975 to 6.1% in 2005. More people suffering from pancreatic cancer are living past the five-year mark. This may be due to a greater understanding about pancreatic cancer and more effective treatment that developed over time.

Data

Table 37.3 Percentage of Pancreatic Cancer Deaths in the United States by Age Group, 2006–2010

Age	Percent of deaths
Under 20	0.0%
20 to 34	0.2%
35 to 44	1.4%
45 to 54	8.0%
55 to 64	19.4%
65 to 74	25.8%
75 to 84	29.5%
Over 84	15.7%

Note: Data takes into account all races and both sexes.

Source: http://seer.cancer.gov/statfacts/html/pancreas.html

Analysis

Table 37.3 shows that the likelihood of contracting and dying from pancreatic cancer increases with age in the United States. Although it is possible for younger people to die from pancreatic cancer, the percentage of deaths for people under the age of 34 is less than 1% and only reaches a significant percentage of 19.4% in the 55–64 age group. The highest percentage of death from pancreatic cancer is 29.5%, found with the 75–84 age group. After age 84, a person's likelihood of dying from pancreatic cancer drops to 15.7%.

DISCUSSION QUESTIONS

1. Pancreatic cancer ranked twelfth in estimated new cases in 2013, but ranked fourth in estimated new deaths that same year. What do you believe makes a cancer more dangerous: more new cases and fewer deaths, or vice versa?

2. Symptoms that indicate pancreatic cancer in its early stages are usually mistaken for other, less serious ailments. Based on the list of symptoms above, what other ailments, illnesses, or conditions might these be mistaken for?
3. The data above indicates that the percentage of deaths from pancreatic cancer in the United States is less than 1% up until a person reaches the age of 34. What makes younger people less susceptible to death than older people when it comes to pancreatic cancer?
4. From 2006 to 2010, pancreatic cancer has killed more men annually than it did women. What are some possible reasons for this gender mortality trend in pancreatic cancer?
5. There are four types of pancreatic cancer, including glucagonoma, insulinoma, islet cell tumor, and VIPoma. Which one of these types of pancreatic cancer do you think is the most fatal for diagnosed patients and why?

38

PRESCRIPTION DRUG USE

INTRODUCTION

Understanding Prescription Drug Use

Prescription drugs are medications that, by law, require any licensed doctor or medical professional—including dentists, optometrists, and clinical pharmacists—to complete and sign a prescription form with the name and dose of the drug on it. Prescription drugs are often referred to simply by their abbreviation "Rx." Used to treat a variety of different illnesses, diseases, and conditions, prescription drugs come in generic or brand name forms—both with the same active ingredient—and are usually either pills, liquids, or gaseous substances that can be swallowed, chewed, injected, or inhaled.

The opposite of a prescription drug is an over-the-counter drug. Although both can usually be obtained in the same pharmacy, over-the-counter drugs do not require a prescription and usually treat illnesses or conditions that do not require immediate medical attention.

Types

Prescription drugs are usually categorized into three groups: opioids, depressants, and stimulants. Opioids are prescribed to relieve pain in cases like surgery recovery or injury trauma. Depressants can slow down and relax the nervous system for patients with anxiety or trouble sleeping. Finally, stimulants increase or augment the processes of the body to treat health issues like asthma, brain disorders, and even obesity.

Some common prescription drugs that fall into one of these three categories of opioids, depressants, and stimulants include:

- Oxycodone
- Hydrocodone
- Codeine
- Methadone
- Benzodiazepines
- Alprazolam
- Eszopiclone
- Dextroamphetamine
- Methylphenidate

These chemical names also have brand names that can be easily recognized by patients and doctors alike. For example, chemical name oxycodone can be called by one of its many brand names, such as OxyContin, Percocet, Roxicodone, or Percodan.

Side Effects

Consuming prescription drugs, even when taken in the correct dosage prescribed, can produce several side effects. Because their appearance is based on the unique reaction of a person's body to the drug in question, they cannot be predicted beforehand. However, any possible side effects—whether they are debilitating or minor—must be listed on the information insert that comes with each prescription drug.

Some of the most common minor side effects of prescription drugs include:

- Rash
- Diarrhea

- Headaches
- Stomachaches
- Dizziness
- Nausea
- Drowsiness
- Constipation

Some of the more severe side effects that occur as a result of taking prescription drugs include:

- Cancer
- Heart attack
- Diabetes
- Death
- Suicidal thoughts
- Paralysis
- Incontinence
- Numbness
- Stroke

Abuse

When a person uses their or another person's prescription drug without a prescription, in a way other than prescribed, or for the feeling they get after they take it, they are abusing a prescription drug. This type of abuse has several short- and long-term consequences, depending on the type of prescription drug. However, a person can not only experience more severe forms of the drug's side effects while they abuse the drug, they can also become vulnerable to seizures and other health issues if they try to stop abusing the drug.

Unfortunately, prescription drug abuse often culminates in prescription drug addiction. Contrary to popular belief, addiction to prescription drugs is just as dangerous as addiction to illicit drugs. Even though prescription drugs are regulated, they can still have very forceful, potentially damaging effects on the body if abused, and especially if abused for a long period of time. These effects are similar to those of even the hardest of illicit drugs, like cocaine or heroin.

DATA AND ANALYSES

Data

Table 38.1 Trends in the Percentage of People Taking Prescription Drugs in the United States, 1999–2008

Year group	Use of 1 or more drugs	Use of 2 or more drugs	Use of 5 or more drugs
1999–2000	43.5%	25.4%	6.3%
2001–2002	46.2%	28.6%	8.3%
2003–2004	47.6%	31.1%	10.2%
2005–2006	46.8%	30.9%	10.1%
2007–2008	48.3%	31.2%	10.7%

Source: http://www.cdc.gov/nchs/data/databriefs/db42.htm

Analysis

Table 38.1 provides an interesting timeline between 1999 and 2008 for prescription drug use in the United States, showing the percentage of people who took one or more, two or more, and five or more drugs in a given two-year group.

In each category, the percentages of people using prescription drugs increased as the years progressed. For example, 43.5% of Americans used one or more prescription drugs from 1999 to 2000 while 48.5% did from 2007 to 2008. People using two or more drugs showed the largest increase in percentage, with 25.4% of users from 1999 to 2000, and 31.2% of users from 2007 to 2008.

Data

Table 38.2 Percentage of Use of at East One Prescription Drug by Gender and Age in the United States, 2007 to 2008

Demographic subgroup	Percentage
Gender	
Male	43.2%
Female	53.3%
Age	
0–11 years old	22.4%
12–19 years old	29.9%
20–59 years old	48.3%
60 years and older	88.4%

Source: http://www.cdc.gov/nchs/data/databriefs/db42.htm

Analysis

Table 38.2 shows the percentage of people in the United States who used at least one prescription drug during 2007 and 2008. The table breaks down the information into gender and age for more detailed data.

In general, during the two-year time frame, more women (53.3%) used at least one prescription drug than men (43.2%) did. Also, older age groups had a higher likelihood of using at least one prescription drug than younger age groups. People aged 60 years and older were those with the highest percentage of prescription drug use, with 88.4%—almost four times that of the 0–11-year-old age group.

Data

Table 38.3 Percentage of Americans Who Take Prescriptions in Relation to Their Access to Health Care Services, 2007–2008

Health care status	Percentage
Have regular health care	52.5%
Do not have regular health care	19.7%
Have health insurance	52.8%
Do not have health insurance	28.5%
Have prescription drug benefit	53.6%
Do not have prescription drug benefit	44.0%

Source: http://www.cdc.gov/nchs/data/databriefs/db42.htm

Analysis

Table 38.3 relates a person's use of prescription drugs to their health care service access—whether or not they have regular health care, health insurance, or a prescription drug benefit.

In the two-year timespan from 2007 to 2008, people in the United States who *did* have health care, health insurance, and a prescription drug benefit had a higher percentage of drug use than those who *did not* have any one of the three health care service options. For example, 52.5% of people who had regular health care used prescription drugs, while 19.7% of those who did not have health care did. Likewise, 52.8% of people who had health insurance and 53.6% of people who had a prescription drug benefit used prescription drugs. This was as opposed to the 28.5% who did not have health insurance and 44.0% who did not have a prescription drug benefit.

DISCUSSION QUESTIONS

1. Although prescription drug use and general drug use may seem like the same concept, they are not the same thing. What are some similarities and differences between the two?

2. According to the data above, more people in the United States are using prescription drugs than they were a decade or so ago. What are some possible reasons for this?

3. In the 1980s, drug companies began marketing drugs to the individual, rather than to doctors. What kind of effect do you think this had on prescription drug use in the United States?

4. Considering the data relating prescription drug use with age, more people use prescription drugs as their age increases. Why does older age logically correlate with increased prescription drug use?

5. Prescription drug use sometimes culminates in prescription drug addiction, especially for teenagers. Why might teens be especially susceptible to this health issue?

39

PROSTATE CANCER

INTRODUCTION

Understanding Prostate Cancer

The prostate is an important gland in the male reproductive system that is key not only in protecting sperm but also in passing urine. Located below the bladder and in front of the bowel, the prostate gland sits in a crucial position that can compromise these and other surrounding organs of the body if it is affected by any illness or disease. Unfortunately, this is often the case. Prostate cancer is one of the most common types of cancer and wreaks havoc on the prostate and its related functions.

Prostate cancer forms when cells in the tissues of the gland become cancerous and begin to attack this very susceptible area of the body. It is worth noting that, just like ovarian cancer can only affect women, prostate cancer can only affect men.

Symptoms

Like most other cancers, the symptoms of prostate cancer are not immediately apparent in its early stages and become more noticeable as the disease progresses. The symptoms of prostate cancer include:

- Difficulty passing urine
- Painful urination

- Weak or interrupted flow or urine
- Frequent urination, especially at night
- Hematuria, or having blood in the urine
- Impotence, or difficulty getting an erection
- Painful ejaculation
- Pain in the hips, pelvis, back, or chest
- Weakness
- Numbness of the legs or feet
- Loss of bladder or bowel control

Diagnosis

Because symptoms of prostate cancer are not immediately apparent, several tests that can be conducted to pinpoint the cancer early on exist. These include the prostate-specific antigen (PSA) test, the digital rectal exam, and the transrectal ultrasound. A PSA test is a blood test that checks for levels of PSA and can help stage or locate the cancer if it is present in the body. During a digital rectal exam, the examining doctor or nurse inserts a lubricated finger into the rectum to check for any cancerous lumps in the prostate. A transrectal ultrasound involves sound waves, echoes, and probes that project a full image of the prostate and check the cancer's density. Recently, researchers have found that semen tests can also improve diagnosis of prostate cancer, aside from these other three tests. The semen test turns up certain biomarkers in the semen sample that indicate cancer.

After any one of these screening tests is conducted and prostate cancer is thought to be detected, a doctor might choose to perform a prostate biopsy and remove a sample of the prostate tissue to examine further. The prostate biopsy is the only certain way to diagnose prostate cancer and is usually performed in conjunction with a transrectal ultrasound.

Risk Factors

Although scientists, doctors, and researchers sometimes clash on the exact causes of prostate cancer, they tend to agree on the risk factors associated with the cancer. The risk factors that increase the chance of contracting prostate cancer include:

- Older age
- Having a family history of prostate cancer
- Inheriting certain gene variations linked to prostate cancer
- Being black or non-Hispanic

- Eating a diet high in red meat, high-fat dairy, and calcium
- Being obese
- Being exposed to toxic combustion substances

Treatment

As with most other cancers, treatment administered by a doctor or medical professional usually depends on the stage of the cancer in relation to the strength of the individual to be treated. Men with prostate cancer have a variety of treatment options, which usually fall into the categories of surgery, radiation therapy, and hormone therapy.

Surgery can entail either a prostatectomy, which completely removes the prostate gland from the body via operation, or a radical prostatectomy, which removes the tissue around the prostate in addition to the gland itself to ensure all cancer is eliminated. Radiation therapy projects rays either externally with a machine or internally with surgically inserted radioactive pellets onto the cancer cells in the prostate and surrounding areas to kill the cells. Finally, hormone therapy cuts off the supply of certain hormones that prostate cancer cells have been found to thrive on.

Aside from these popular treatments, there are also alternative treatments that some men have opted to undergo. These include cell-freezing cryotherapy, chemotherapy, immune system-based biological therapy, and high-intensity focused ultrasound.

DATA AND ANALYSES

Data

Table 39.1 Estimated New Cases and Death for Common Types of Cancer in the United States, 2014

Common types of cancer	Estimated new cases 2014	Estimated deaths 2014
Prostate cancer	233,000	29,480
Breast cancer	232,670	40,000
Lung and bronchus cancer	224,210	159,260
Colon and rectum cancer	136,830	50,310
Melanoma of the skin	76,100	9,710
Bladder cancer	74,690	15,580
Non-Hodgkin lymphoma	70,800	18,990
Kidney and renal pelvis cancer	63,920	13,860
Thyroid cancer	62,980	1,890
Endometrial cancer	52,630	8,590

Source: http://seer.cancer.gov/statfacts/html/prost.html

Analysis

Table 39.1, The table above indicates the most common types of cancer and their projected new cases and deaths for 2014 in the United States. Because prostate cancer is one of the most common types of cancer, it is no surprise that it tops the list with 233,000 estimated new cases for 2014. However, it does not have the highest number of estimated death for 2014. In fact, it is estimated that prostate cancer will the cause of 29,480 deaths in 2014, the fourth largest number of estimated deaths in the list behind lung and bronchus cancer (159,260 estimated deaths), colon and rectum cancer (50,310 estimated deaths), and breast cancer (40,000 estimated deaths).

Data

Table 39.2 Percent of New Cases of Prostate Cancer in the United States by Age Group, 2007–2011

Age	Percentage
<20 years old	0.0%
20–34 years old	0.0%
35–44 years old	0.6%
45–54 years old	9.7%
55–64 years old	32.7%
65–74 years old	36.3%
75–84 years old	16.8%
>84 years old	3.8%

Note: Data takes into account men of all races.

Source: http://seer.cancer.gov/statfacts/html/prost.html

Analysis

Table 39.2 demonstrates the percentage of new cases of prostate cancer among men of different ages in the United States. It is worth noting that because prostate cancer is a sex-specific cancer, women are not included in the data. In the four-year span from 2007 to 2011, it is clear that as men aged, the percentage of new cases of prostate cancer increased significantly, peaking at the 65–74 age group. In fact, the median age at diagnosis for prostate cancer is 66 years old. In all subsequent age groups, the percentage of new cases of prostate cancer begins to decrease. For example, in the >84 age group, the percentage of new cases is a mere 3.8%.

Data

Table 39.3 Number of New Cases of Prostate Cancer in the United States by Race and Ethnicity, 2007–2011

Race/ethnicity	Number
All races	147.8
White	139.9
Black	223.9
Asian/Pacific Islander	79.3
American Indian/Alaska Native	71.5
Hispanic	122.6
Non-Hispanic	151.5

Note: Numbers are per 100,000 men.

Source: http://seer.cancer.gov/statfacts/html/prost.html

Analysis

Table 39.3 indicates the number of new cases of prostate cancer in the United States based on a man's race and ethnicity. It is worth noting that because prostate cancer is a sex-specific cancer, women are not included in the table data. In the four-year span from 2007 to 2011, it was found that there were significantly more new cases of prostate cancer—223.9 new cases—among black men than any other race or ethnicity. This is an extremely significant number, especially when compared to American Indian and Alaska Native men. These groups had the lowest number of new cases compared to the other races and ethnicities listed, with 71.5 new cases. Interestingly, black men are also twice as likely to die as a result of prostate cancer as white men.

DISCUSSION QUESTIONS

1. Because only men can contract it, prostate cancer is a sex-specific cancer. Can you think of any other sex-specific cancers that affect men and women?
2. According to the data above, prostate cancer is most frequently diagnosed among men in the 65–74 age range, after which point the percentage of new cases begins to fall. What are some possible reasons for this?
3. Prostate cancer is the most common type of cancer in men. Why do you think this area of the male reproductive system is so susceptible to cancer than other parts of the male body?

4. One of the symptoms of prostate cancer is numbness in the legs or feet. How can cancer in the prostate have an effect on these areas of the body instead of arms and hands?
5. Based on the data above, some races and ethnicities are more susceptible to prostate cancer than others. For example, black men have significantly higher numbers of new cases than all other races and ethnicities. Why do you think this is?

40

SKIN CANCER

INTRODUCTION

Skin cancer is the most common cancer in the United States. There are three main different types of skin cancer: basal cell skin cancer, squamous cell skin cancer, and melanoma.

Basal cell skin cancer is skin cancer that commences in the basal cell layer of the skin. Typically, basal cell skin cancer develops in locations that have been subject to sun exposure, such as the skin, the most common place to find basal cell skin cancer. Basal cell skin cancer is the most common type of skin cancer in people with fair skin.

Squamous cell skin cancer is skin cancer that begins in squamous cells. It is the most common type of skin cancer for people with dark skin and, in such individuals, this type of cancer is usually found in places that are not in the sun. By contrast, in people with fair skin, squamous cell skin cancer usually occurs on parts of the skin that have been subject to sun exposure.

Melanoma is a disease in which malignant cells form in the skin cells called melanocytes. Melanocytes, which make melanin, are found throughout the lower part of the epidermis. Melanoma can occur on any skin surface. However, there are gender-based differences in where it typically does appear. In men, melanoma is typically found on the skin on the head, on the neck, or between the shoulders and the hips. In women, melanoma is often found on the skin on the lower legs or between the shoulders and the hips.

Melanoma is the deadliest form of skin cancer is melanoma. In 2010 (the most recent year numbers are available) 61,061 people in the United States were diagnosed with melanomas of the skin, including 35,248 men and 25,813 women.

Risk Factors

While anyone can get skin cancer, some people are at higher risk for it than others. Some general risk factors for developing skin cancer are:

- Having a fair complexion natural
- Having a personal or family history of skin cancer
- A personal history of skin cancer
- Exposure to the sun through work and play
- A history of sunburns, particularly sunburns early in life
- A history of indoor tanning
- Skin that burns, freckles, reddens easily, or becomes painful in the sun
- Blue or green eyes
- Blond or red hair
- Certain types and a large number of moles

The most preventable cause of skin cancer is exposure to ultraviolet light, whether from the sun or from artificial sources such as tanning beds.

Symptoms

Skin cancer is typically first observed through changes in the skin. While the appearance of skin cancers can vary considerably, individuals who are concerned about the prospects of skin cancer are advised to evaluate the change in their skin using the "ABCDEs of melanoma":

- Asymmetry: Does the mole or spot have an irregular shape with two parts that look very different?
- Border: Is the border irregular or jagged?
- Color: Is the color uneven?
- Diameter: Is the mole or spot larger than the size of a pea?
- Evolving: Has the mole or spot changed during the past few weeks or months?

An individual who experiences new skin growths, observe a sore that does not heal, notices a change in an old growth, or notices a skin condition that meets any of the ABCDEs of melanoma should consult his or her physician for an examination of the skin condition. If the physician expects that the skin condition may be cancerous, the physician may order a biopsy of the skin. The biopsy will confirm whether or not skin cancer exists.

Treatment

Most skin cancers can be cured if found and treated early. Treatment for skin cancer depends upon various factors, including the type and stage of the disease, the size and place of the tumor, and one's overall health. In most cases, the skin cancer will be removed with surgery. In some cases, chemotherapy, photodynamic therapy, or radiation therapy may also be needed.

DATA AND ANALYSES

Data

Table 40.1 Melanoma of the Skin Incidence Rates* by State, 2010

Interval	States
7.6 to 17.5	Alaska, Arizona, District of Columbia, Florida, Illinois, Louisiana, Mississippi, Missouri, Nebraska, Nevada, New York, Oklahoma, Texas, and Virginia
17.6 to 21.0	California, Indiana, Massachusetts, Michigan, New Jersey, New Mexico, Ohio, Pennsylvania, South Dakota, West Virginia, and Wisconsin
21.1 to 22.4	Alabama, Colorado, Georgia, Hawaii, Kansas, Maine, Maryland, North Carolina, North Dakota, Rhode Island, South Carolina, and Tennessee
22.5 to 33.4	Connecticut, Delaware, Idaho, Iowa, Kentucky, Montana, New Hampshire, Oregon, Utah, Vermont, Washington, and Wyoming
Data not available‡	Arkansas and Minnesota

*Rates are per 100,000 and are age-adjusted to the 2000 U.S. standard population.
‡Rates are not shown if the state did not meet USCS publication criteria or if the state did not submit data to CDC.
Source: U.S. Cancer Statistics Working Group. 2013. "United States cancer statistics: 1999–2010 incidence and mortality web-based report." Department of Health and Human Services, Centers for Disease Control and Prevention, and National Cancer Institute. Retrieved from: http://www.cdc.gov/uscs

Analysis

In the United States, the rate of getting melanoma varies from state to state. A demonstrated in Table 40.1, the highest rates of skin cancer are in Connecticut, Delaware, Idaho, Iowa, Kentucky, Montana, New Hampshire, Oregon, Utah, Vermont, Washington, and Wyoming. Because sun exposure is a major factor in the development of melanoma, one might expect high rates of melanoma in states that have a lot of sunshine and in which individuals spend a lot of time at the beach or otherwise engaging in outdoor activities where there skin is exposed to the sun. However, Florida and Arizona actually were in the group of states with the lowest rates of melanoma, California was in the group of states with the second lowest incidence of melanoma, and Hawaii was in the group of states with the third lowest incidence of melanoma.

Data

Table 40.2 Melanoma of the Skin Death Rates* by State, 2010

Interval	States
1.8 to 2.5	Georgia, Hawaii, Illinois, Louisiana, Maryland, Michigan, Mississippi, Montana, New Hampshire, New Jersey, New York, South Carolina, and South Dakota
2.6 to 2.8	Alabama, California, Connecticut, Delaware, Florida, Iowa, Kansas, Minnesota, Nebraska, Nevada, Rhode Island, and Texas
2.9 to 3.1	Alaska, Arizona, Arkansas, Indiana, Maine, Massachusetts, New Mexico, North Carolina, Pennsylvania, Virginia, Washington, Wisconsin, and Wyoming
3.2 to 3.7	Colorado, Idaho, Kentucky, Missouri, Ohio, Oklahoma, Oregon, Tennessee, Utah, Vermont, and West Virginia
Data not available‡	District of Columbia and North Dakota

*Rates are per 100,000 and are age-adjusted to the 2000 U.S. standard population.
‡Rates are suppressed if fewer than 16 deaths were reported by a state.
Source: U.S. Cancer Statistics Working Group. 2013. "United States cancer statistics: 1999–2010.incidence and mortality web-based report." Department of Health and Human Services, Centers for Disease Control and Prevention, and National Cancer Institute. Retrieved from: http://www.cdc.gov/uscs

Analysis

Just as the incidence rates of melanoma vary from state to state so do the rates of dying from melanoma. Understanding differences in melanoma death rates from state to state can be helpful to researchers trying to reduce the risks of dying from melanoma.

Data

Table 40.3 Five-year Relative Survival Rates From Skin Cancer

Year	1975	1980	1985	1989	1993	1997	2001	2005
5-year relative survival	81.9%	83.8%	86.1%	87.6%	90.2%	89.8%	92.1%	93.1%

Source: http://seer.cancer.gov/statfacts/html/melan.html

Analysis

Skin cancer survival rates have been improving. In 1975, the five-year relative survival rate for skin cancer was 81.9%. By 2005, the survival rate had increased to 93.1%. These trends are consistent with cancer more generally. Statistics show that cancer patients are living longer lives and enjoying a better quality of life. Still, despite these advances, improvements are still needed in skin cancer prevention, detection, and treatments.

DISCUSSION QUESTIONS

1. The most preventable cause of skin cancer is exposure to ultraviolet (UV) light, either from the sun or from artificial sources such as tanning beds. Given the skin cancer risks posed by tanning beds, do you believe that tanning salons should be prohibited? Why or why not?
2. As demonstrated in Tables 40.2 and 40.3, melanoma incidence and death rates vary from state to state. What do you think are some of the reasons for these differences?
3. Many skin cancers can be prevented through changes in behaviors (such as protecting one's skin from sun exposure) and yet people continue to develop breast cancer. What more can be done to raise public awareness of the risks of skin cancer and the need to commit to take preventative measures?
4. Table 40.3 shows that over the past 20 years there has been an increase in melanoma survival rates. What are some possible factors that may have influenced the increased survival rates?

41

SMOKING AND TOBACCO USE

INTRODUCTION

Understanding Smoking and Tobacco Use

Smoking and tobacco use harms nearly every organ of the body and can cause many serious diseases, reducing the overall health of everyone who smokes. Tobacco smoke contains over sixty known cancer-causing chemicals and various other harmful substances. Nicotine is the addictive chemical in tobacco, causing a temporary rush of adrenaline when inhaled or absorbed in the bloodstream. Reaching the brain within ten seconds of entering the body, nicotine also causes an increase of the neurotransmitter dopamine, which improves mood and increases feelings of pleasure. Furthermore, nicotine stimulates the areas of the brain associated with reward and pleasure. However, the feelings provided by nicotine fade quickly and lead to fatigue, as well as a craving for more nicotine, tempting individuals to use tobacco again in order to keep the pleasurable feeling. Over time, individuals can build up a tolerance to nicotine; therefore, repeated use of tobacco can cause physical and psychological addiction.

While smoking cigarettes and chewing tobacco are the most common ways that individuals use tobacco, other methods of tobacco use include pipes, cigars, and snuff.

Symptoms

Some individuals may smoke recreationally or only occasionally; however, tobacco use is very addictive. If an individual cannot stop smoking or chewing tobacco despite repeated attempts to quit, then they are considered to be addicted. While smoking is legal and can be done in public, some smokers, such as teenagers, try to hide their tobacco use. Some physical signs of tobacco use include nicotine-stained brown fingers and teeth, premature wrinkles, smell of smoke on clothes, a deep cough, and a raspy voice.

Other signs of addiction include having to smoke or chew after every meal or after long periods without using, needing tobacco products to feel normal, turning toward tobacco products during times of emotional distress, giving up activities or events where smoking is prohibited, continuing to smoke despite health problems, and experiencing withdrawal symptoms when trying to quit, such as shaky hands, sweating, irritability, or increased heart rate.

Additionally, medical professionals should be contacted if a tobacco user notices any of these symptoms: chest pain, shortness of breath, persistent cough, coughing up blood, frequent colds, persistently hoarse voice, difficulty or painful swallowing, change in exercise abilities, sudden weakness of one side of the face or body, unexplained weight loss, persistent abdominal pain, or blood in the urine. These symptoms are just a few signs that the tobacco use has caused a serious health condition.

Risk Factors

There are many factors that may cause an individual to start smoking. Among adolescents, exposure and susceptibility to tobacco advertising and peer pressure can increase the risk of tobacco use. Specifically, children whose parents and friends smoke are at a higher risk of developing a tobacco addiction. Additionally, characteristics such as stress, difficult living environments, and low self-esteem can also cause adolescents to begin smoking.

There are also risk factors that are related to tobacco addiction. Smoking early in adolescence relates to higher risks of tobacco addiction, as well as genetics. Over twelve different genes that an individual inherits plays a role in how their brain reacts to nicotine and their likelihood of getting addicted. Individuals who suffer from mental illnesses and substance use are also at a higher risk of becoming nicotine dependent.

Increased Health Risks

According to the Centers for Disease Control and Prevention, smoking is the leading preventable cause of death in the United States. Smoking greatly increases the risk of heart disease, stroke, and lung cancer. Cardiovascular disease results from damaged blood vessels, as smoking makes them thicken, increases heart rate and blood pressure, and allows blood clots to form. A stroke occurs when blood clots block the blood flow to the brain, or when a blood vessel in or around the brain bursts. Smoking can also cause lung disease by damaging an individual's airways and the small air sacs in the lungs, known as alveoli. Furthermore, in addition to lung cancer, smoking can cause cancer almost anywhere in the body, including the bladder, blood, cervix, colon and rectum, esophagus, kidney, larynx, live, oropharynx, pancreas, and stomach.

Smoking can also affect an individual's general health. Individuals who smoke have an increased risk of developing lower bone density, unhealthy teeth and gums, cataracts, age-related macular degeneration, type 2 diabetes mellitus, inflammation, suppressed immune functioning, and rheumatoid arthritis. Specifically in females, smoking may decrease the chances of getting pregnant and negatively affect their baby's health. Infertility can also occur in males, as smoking affects their sperm.

Furthermore, smoking can even affect individuals who do not smoke, but live with someone who does. Secondhand smoke can put nonsmokers at a higher risk of developing lung cancer and heart disease. Children are especially affected, as secondhand smoke can lead to sudden infant death syndrome, asthma, ear infections, and colds.

Seeking Help to Quit

Quitting smoking and tobacco use can immediately improve an individual's overall health, lower their risk of smoking-related diseases, and add years to their life. However, the addictive qualities of tobacco make it very hard to quit. Even after nicotine cravings have subsided, individuals may have trouble breaking their behavioral rituals or routines that were associated with smoking. Individuals who are trying to quit smoking or chewing tobacco have several treatment options. Often a combination of treatment methods will help individuals successfully quit smoking and tobacco use and prevent relapse.

The patch is a nicotine replacement therapy that involves placing a small sticker on the arm or back, which delivers low levels of nicotine to the body to help gradually reduce cravings. Similarly, nicotine gum or lozenges may be used for individuals who crave the oral fixation associated with smoking or chewing. Other forms of treatment that help regulate nicotine cravings include using a nicotine nasal spray or nicotine inhaler, or certain antidepressants or antihypertensive drugs.

Some individuals may choose to seek psychological or behavioral treatments in addition to or in replace of nicotine replacement therapy. Hypnotherapy, group therapy, cognitive-behavioral therapy, and neurolinguistic programming are all options. Altering lifestyle habits may also help prevent relapse, including exercising or finding a hobby to do when cravings start, or avoiding situations where there will be tobacco.

DATA AND ANALYSES

Data

Table 41.1 Percentage of Individuals Who Were Current Cigarette Smokers by Gender and Age: United States, 2005 and 2012

Age	Male smokers in 2005	Male smokers in 2012	Female smokers in 2005	Female smokers in 2012
18–24 years	28.0%	20.1%	20.7%	14.5%
25–44 years	26.8%	25.4%	21.4%	17.8%
45–64 years	25.2%	20.2%	18.8%	18.9%
65 years and older	8.9%	10.6%	8.3%	7.5%

Source: Agaku, I.T., Dube, S.R., & King, B.A. 2014. "Current cigarette smoking among adults—United States, 2005–2012." Centers for Disease Control and Prevention. Retrieved from: http://www.cdc.gov/mmwr/preview/mmwrhtml/mm6302a2. htm?s_cid=mm6302a2_w

Analysis

More than 42 million adults in the United States were reported cigarette smokers during 2012. Fortunately, overall smoking prevalence has decreased from 20.9% in 2005 to 18.1% in 2012. The data above examines the prevalence of smokers based on gender and age. The largest population of smokers in 2012 were males aged 25–44 years old.

Table 41.1 presents that there is a greater number of males that smoke than females for all age group categories. The overall prevalence of male smokers in 2012 was 20.5%, while only 15.8% of females smoked. For both genders, the greatest decrease between 2005 and 2012 was seen in individuals aged 18 to 24 years old. Further research can determine whether this decline is related to the availability of new tobacco products. Additionally, while most age groups presented a decrease in smoking between 2005 and 2012, two age groups presented an increase. Males aged 65 and older showed a slight increase in smoking, as well as females aged 45–64. Further research can also determine the causes for these slight increases and how to decrease the rates.

Data

Table 41.2 Percentage of Individuals Who Were Current Cigarette Smokers by Gender and Race/ethnicity: United States, 2005 and 2012

Race/ethnicity	Male smokers in 2005	Male smokers in 2012	Female smokers in 2005	Female smokers in 2012
White	24.0%	21.1%	20.0%	18.4%
Black	26.7%	22.1%	17.3%	14.8%
Hispanic	21.1%	17.2%	11.1%	7.8%
American Indian/ Alaska Native	37.5%	25.5%	26.8%	18.7%
Asian	20.6%	16.7%	6.1%	5.5%
Multiple race	26.1%	28.6%	23.5%	23.9%

Source: Agaku, I.T., Dube, S.R., & King, B.A. 2014. "Current cigarette smoking among adults—United States, 2005–2012." Centers for Disease Control and Prevention. Retrieved from: http://www.cdc.gov/mmwr/preview/mmwrhtml/mm6302a2. htm?s_cid=mm6302a2_w

Analysis

Table 41.2 further examines the rates of cigarette smokers by gender and race/ethnicity between the years of 2005 and 2012. For all race/ethnicities besides multiple race individuals, smoking rates declined between the years 2005 and 2012. Similar to the data above, males presented higher smoking rates than females.

Specifically, multiple race individuals presented slight increases in smoking rates between 2005 and 2012, as well as the highest over-all rates. American Indian/Alaska Native individuals presented high smoking rates as well. For males, blacks presented the next highest smoking rate, followed by whites; however, the trend was opposite for females, as 18.4% of white females smoked in 2012, fol-lowed by only 14.8% of black females.

In both genders, American Indian/Alaska Natives presented the greatest decrease in smokers from 2005 to 2012. Further research can determine why their race/ethnicity showed the greatest decline and how other race/ethnicities can decrease their rates as well.

Data

Table 41.3 Estimated Annual Cigarette Smoking-related Mortality Among Smokers Aged 35 Years and Older: United States, 2005–2009

Disease	Total deaths
Cancer	163,700
Cardiovascular diseases and metabolic diseases	160,000
Respiratory diseases	113,100
Perinatal conditions	1,013
Residential fires	620
Secondhand smoke	41,284
Total attributable deaths	480,317

Source: http://www.cdc.gov/tobacco/data_statistics/fact_sheets/health_effects/tobacco_related_mortality/

Analysis

Tobacco use is the leading preventable cause of death in the United States. Overall, mortality rates are about three times higher in smokers than nonsmokers. The major causes of cigarette-smoking related mortality are diseases, including cancers, cardiovascular and metabolic diseases, and respiratory diseases. Following these causes, secondhand smoke, perinatal conditions, and residential fires are also smoking-related causes of mortality.

Cancer is the greatest cause of smoking-related mortality. Specifi-cally, 127,700 smokers die from lung cancer, while 36,000 smokers die from other cancers. Of cardiovascular and metabolic diseases, the most smokers die from coronary heart disease, followed by other forms of heart disease, cerebrovascular disease, other vascu-lar diseases, and diabetes mellitus. Of respiratory diseases, chronic obstructive pulmonary disease (COPD) accounts for 100,600 deaths and includes emphysema, bronchitis, and chronic airway obstruction. Of secondhand smoke deaths, coronary heart disease accounts for 33,951 deaths, while lung cancer accounts for 7,333 deaths. Further research can examine the relationship between smoking and these life-threatening diseases in order to decrease mortality rates.

DISCUSSION QUESTIONS

1. Why was the greatest decrease in cigarette smoking seen among 18–24-year-olds? Are these individuals using other forms of tobacco instead?
2. Why are there more reported male smokers than females? How can both genders' smoking rates be decreased?
3. Why do multiple race and American Indian/Alaska Natives present the highest smoking rates? Do socioeconomic factors affect these rates?
4. How can tobacco use be decreased in the United States? How much of an impact will a decrease in smoking rates have on overall morbidity rates?
5. Can mortality from secondhand smoke be decreased even if there is no change in smoking rates? How can smokers be educated about the effects on not only their body, but on non-smokers around them as well?

42

STDs

INTRODUCTION

Understanding Sexually Transmitted Diseases

Sexually transmitted diseases (STDs), also referred to as sexually transmitted infections, are typically acquired through sexual contact, as the organisms that carry STDs pass from person to person via blood, semen, vaginal fluids, or other body fluids. However, some STDs can be nonsexually transmitted. Nonsexual transmission occurs through blood transfusions, shared needles, or a mother passing the disease on to an infant during pregnancy. There are over 20 types of STDs. Different STDs have specific causes, such as gonorrhea, syphilis, and chlamydia, which are caused by bacteria; trichomoniasis, which is caused by parasites; and, human papillomavirus, genital herpes, and HIV, which are caused by viruses.

Symptoms

Many STDs do not present any symptoms, so individuals can be unaware that they are carrying a disease until complications arise or a sexual partner is diagnosed. Yet, STDs can present a range of symptoms, appearing a few days up to a few years after exposure. Common symptoms of STDs include:

- Sores or bumps on the genitals, in the oral area, or in the rectal area
- Pain or burning during urination
- Vaginal discharge
- Unusual vaginal bleeding
- Sore, swollen lymph nodes, usually in the groin
- Lower abdominal pain
- Rash over the abdomen, hands, or feet

The progression of undiagnosed STDs can eventually lead to serious complications, including arthritis, pelvic inflammatory disease, infertility, cervical and other cancers, birth defects from maternal-fetal transmission, and other complications.

Diagnosis

Individuals should seek medical attention if they are sexually active and believe they have contracted a STD or if they are presenting symptoms of a STD. Routine general STD screening tests should be completed upon becoming sexually active. If sexual history and present symptoms suggest that an individual has a STD, laboratory tests can determine the type and cause of the STD. Blood tests are often used to diagnose HIV and later stages of syphilis. Fluid samples are often used to diagnose STDs that produce genital sores or discharge, including many bacterial and viral STDs. Additionally, urine samples may be used to detect other STDs.

Risk Factors

Anyone who is sexually active increases their risk of contracting a STD. Additional factors that can increase the risk of acquiring STDs are:

- Having unprotected sex: If a partner is infected, having sex without a condom allows for easier transmission of STDs during vaginal or anal penetration. Improper use of condoms also increases the risk of STDs.
- Having sex with multiple partners: The more individuals that one has sex with, the greater their chance of developing STDs.

- Having a history of STDs: Having a previous STD increases the risk of contracting another STD. Additionally, reinfection may occur.
- Abusing alcohol or drugs: Substance abuse inhibits judgment, which may increase the risk of engaging with more sexual partners. Additionally, injecting drugs via needles increases the risk of serious STDs such as HIV, hepatitis B, and hepatitis C.
- Being an adolescent female: Cells in the cervix are still growing and changing in adolescent females, putting them at a higher risk of acquiring STDs. Females also face more serious health problems if affected with STDs.
- Not receiving vaccinations: Vaccinations can prevent human papillomavirus, hepatitis A, and hepatitis B, which are all viral infections that can cause cancer. If an individual is not vaccinated before sexual exposure, they increase the risk of STDs.

STDs can travel quickly in communities that have overlapping sexual partners. The Centers for Disease Control and Prevention found that these communities often include young individuals, males who have sex with males, and minorities, as these groups tend to seek sexual partners with similar ages, locations, and backgrounds.

Treatment

Some STDs may resolve in a few weeks without treatment; however, diseases can also recur or lead to later complications, which is why it is important to seek treatment if diagnosed. Typically, STDs caused by bacteria are the easiest to treat. STDs caused by viruses cannot always be cured, yet they can be controlled. Options for treatment include antibiotics and antiviral drugs.

Antibiotics can often cure many STDs caused by bacteria and parasites, such as gonorrhea, syphilis, chlamydia, and trichomoniasis. It is important to follow through with treatment, even though a single dose can often result in a cure. Additionally, it is important to abstain from sex until treatment is completed.

Antiviral drugs are used to control STDs caused by viruses. For example, daily suppressive therapy and antiviral drugs decrease the recurrence of herpes. However, since antiviral drugs are not a complete cure, individuals may still transmit the STD to sexual partners at any time. Antiviral drugs also help control HIV. Antiviral drugs should be taken as soon as possible in order to decrease the presence of symptoms.

DATA AND ANALYSES

Data

Table 42.1 Estimated Number of New Sexually Transmitted Diseases Divided by Age Group Population: United States, 2008

Type of STD	Number of 15–24 year olds infected	Prevalence (%) in 15–24 year olds	Number of 25+ year olds infected	Prevalence (%) in 25+ year olds	Total estimated number of new cases
Hepatitis B	1,520	8%	17,480	92%	19,000
Syphilis	11,080	20%	44,320	80%	55,400
HIV*	—	—	—	—	41,400
HSV-2	34,920	45%	741,080	55%	776,000
Gonorrhea	574,000	70%	246,000	30%	820,000
Trichomoniasis	141,700	13%	948,300	87%	1,090,000
Chlamydia	1,801,800	63%	1,058,200	37%	2,860,000
HPV	6,909,000	49%	7,191,000	51%	14,100,000

*Incidences for HIV were not able to be calculated by age for this analysis.

Source: Centers for Disease Control and Prevention. 2013. "Incidence, prevalence, and cost of sexually transmitted infections in the United States." Retrieved from: http://www.cdc.gov/std/stats/sti-estimates-fact-sheet-feb-2013.pdf

Analysis

The Centers for Disease Control and Prevention estimated that there were 110,197,000 STDs in the United States during 2008, a total that includes both new and existing infections. There were eight STDs that proved to be the most common: hepatitis B, syphilis, human immunodeficiency virus (HIV), herpes simplex virus type 2 (HSV-2), gonorrhea, trichomoniasis, chlamydia, and human papillomavirus (HPV). Of the total STDs, 19,738,800 were newly contracted during 2008. By examining the new STD cases based on age, results showed that young people ages 15–24 presented half of all new STDs, even though they only represent 25% of the sexually active population.

Table 42.1 shows that HPV accounts for the majority of newly acquired STDs, followed by chlamydia and trichomoniasis. Ninety percent of HPV infections go away on their own within two years, though they can eventually lead to serious complications like cervical cancer. Additionally, the subsequent prevalent infections including chlamydia, trichomoniasis and gonorrhea are easily treated and cured upon early diagnosis; however, these STDs commonly go undetected because they do not present any symptoms. Therefore, there may be even higher rates of these diseases that go undiagnosed. These diseases can also have serious health effects if left untreated, especially for females who can become infertile or be at risk for life-threatening ectopic pregnancies. In conclusion, the data presented above shows the importance of educating young individuals on practicing safe sex. Since young individuals account for half of all newly acquired STDs, reducing the rates of STDs in their age-group population will significantly decrease the total amount of STDs in the United States.

Data

Table 42.2 Reported Chlamydia and Gonorrhea Infections by Age Group Population: United States, 2011

Age-group population	Reported gonorrhea cases	Prevalence (%) of gonorrhea cases	Reported chlamydia cases	Prevalence (%) of chlamydia cases
0–14 year olds	3,218.49	1	14,127.91	1
15–19 year olds	86,899.23	27	452,093.12	32
20–24 year olds	112,647.15	35	536,860.58	38
25–29 year olds	54,714.33	17	211,918.65	15
30–39 year olds	41,840.37	13	127,151.19	9
40+ year olds	22,529.43	7	42,383.73	3
All ages	321,849	—	1,412,791	—

Source: Centers for Disease Control and Prevention. 2013. "STD trends in the United States." Retrieved from: http://www.cdc.gov/std/stats11/trends-2011.pdf

Analysis

Supporting the data presented in Table 42.1, Table 42.2 presents STD prevalence based on age-group population from the United States in 2011. The table further examined the differences in STD prevalence between age-group populations focusing solely on gonorrhea and chlamydia cases. The data confirms that reported gonorrhea and chlamydia rates are highest in Americans between the ages of 15 and 24, followed by 25–29-year-olds. Since there are so many STD cases in younger individuals, preventative measures should be created and adapted to help decrease overall STD prevalence.

Data

Table 42.3 Reported STD Infections by Gender: United States, 2011

Type of STD	Number of females affected	Number of males affected	Number of cases with unreported gender
Chancroid	4	4	—
Chlamydia	1,018,552	389,970	4,269
Gonorrhea	171,005	149,835	1,009
Syphilis	9,712	36,625	65
All STDs Listed	1,199,273	576,434	5,343

Source: Centers for Disease Control and Prevention. 2012. "Sexually transmitted disease surveillance 2011." Retrieved from: http://wonder.cdc.gov/wonder/help/STD/STDSurv2011.pdf

Analysis

Table 42.3 examines the 2011 reported STD infections in the United States categorized by prevalence in genders. Examining reported cases of chancroid, chlamydia, gonorrhea, and syphilis, the data shows that females account for 67.34% of these STDs, while males only account for 32.36% of the STDs listed. These results need to be addressed due to the fact that females often acquire more severe medical complications from STDs, especially those that go undiagnosed. However, the results do support the stated risk factor for females, who are at a high risk of acquiring STDs during the adolescent years when the cells in their cervix are still growing. As young individuals aged 15–24 are accounting for half of all new STDs, it is important to address this gender difference in order to decrease the prevalence of all STDs.

DISCUSSION QUESTIONS

1. Why do 15- to 24-year-olds account for half of all newly acquired STDs when they make up only a quarter of the entire sexually active population? What preventative and educational measures can be taken to lower the prevalence of STDs in this age group?
2. What social, environmental, psychological, and biological factors are related to reported STD cases? Do these certain factors appear as additional risk factors for acquiring STDs?
3. Why are gonorrhea and chlamydia so prevalent in young individuals? Do these diseases transmit easier? If so, what additional ways can they be prevented?

4. What other reasons explain why females acquire more STDs than males? Do social, environmental, psychological, or biological factors play a role?
5. Why do STDs often cause more severe complications in females? How can these complications be addressed and prevented?

43

STRESS

INTRODUCTION

Understanding Stress

Stress is the brain's response to any demand, according to the National Institute of Mental Health. A variety of occurrences can trigger this response, especially lifestyle changes. Whether changes are positive or negative, short term or long term, major, or minor, all have an impact on stress level. These changes can occur during daily tasks or less frequently. During stressful times, the nervous system releases stress hormones including adrenaline and cortisol, preparing the body for "fight or flight." The release of these hormones increases physical strength and stamina, reaction time, and focus; however, if stress persists, it can lead to negative physical, emotional, and behavioral symptoms that impact individual's lives.

Three types of stress are identified, including: routine stress that relates to daily responsibilities, pressures of work, and family relations; traumatic stress, which occurs during major events such as car accidents, war, assault, or natural disasters; and stress that occurs due to a sudden negative change such as divorce, illness, or losing a job. The body responds differently depending on which type of stress is experienced.

Symptoms

In stressful situations, the body responds with functions that are geared towards survival and will subside after the stress is lifted. Some common symptoms that occur during stressful times include:

- Quickened pulse
- Faster breathing
- Tense muscles

However, in long term, stress responses can suppress functions that are not required for immediate survival. This can lead to a lowered immunity and abnormal functioning of the digestive, excretory, and reproductive systems. When stress is constant or occurs for too long, these problems may occur. Often undetectable at first, individuals experience longer-term symptoms of stress in different ways. Common long-term symptoms of stress may affect an individual's body are:

- Physical symptoms: Headaches, muscle tension, chest pain, fatigue, change in sex drive, upset stomach, or sleep problems
- Emotional symptoms: Anxiety, restlessness, lack of motivation, lack of concentration, irritability or anger, and depression
- Behavioral symptoms: Changes in appetite, drug or alcohol abuse, social withdrawal, and the development of nervous habits such as nail biting or pacing

Additionally, chronic stress can lead to other health complications such as diabetes, high blood pressure, heart disease, or viral infections such as the flu or common cold.

Risk Factors

Since there are various causes and types of stress, there are many factors that can increase an individual's susceptibility to stress. Typically, an accumulation of stressful situations and persistent stress increase the risk of developing negative stress reactions.

Individuals will respond differently to stress depending on how they were raised, their personality traits, genetic factors, and if they have certain immune-regulated diseases, which weaken stress responses. Various types of individuals are at a higher risk of experiencing stress and its negative symptoms, including: the elderly; undereducated, unemployed, or impoverished individuals; divorcees or widows; females, specifically working mothers; individuals who are isolated or lonely; and individuals who have been discriminated against, abused, or experienced another sort of trauma. Additionally, children who are raised in stressful environments with parents that cannot properly cope with their own stress tend to be more vulnerable to stress as they age.

Work environments can be stressful, posing certain factors that increase stress levels, such as: Having little power in decisions that affect one's responsibilities; being held to unreasonable demands or performance standards; lacking effective communication among coworkers; lacking job security; working the night shift or long hours; spending time away from the home and family; and not earning proper payment for responsibilities.

Many additional factors can increase the risk of stress, including other medical conditions, lack of social support, etc. It is important to recognize which factors are contributing to an individual's stress in order to help prevent and maintain stress levels.

Diagnosis

Everyone reacts differently to stress, with some people not recognizing stress symptoms until days after stressful situations have occurred or persisted. It is important to recognize the possible symptoms of stress so that individuals can be aware of the cause of their stress and manage it on their own with healthy coping skills. Individuals can track their stress by keeping a log of their symptoms, lifestyle changes, and any other factors that they believe may be contributing to their stress.

While there is no specific test that diagnoses stress, medical professionals can also diagnose stress based on symptoms that individuals present, asking about family history, and asking about any lifestyle changes that may have occurred. Occasionally, blood tests, urine tests, and general health assessments may also be administered by a medical professional in order to check for underlying health conditions that may be causing the stress or health complications that may have arisen from the stress.

Treatment

Stress can be reduced or alleviated in many different ways; however, treatment depends on the symptoms, cause, and type of stress.

Seeking medical attention and therapy may be helpful for individuals who are overwhelmed, feeling that they cannot cope with their stress, or are coping with their stress in harmful ways, such as abusing drugs or alcohol. Additionally, seeking medical attention will help identify and cure health problems that are occurring alongside or because of the stress.

Individually, stress can be recognized by becoming aware of the body's responses. Subsequently, stress levels can be prevented and maintained by simple actions such as seeking emotional support from loved ones or community organizations, setting appropriate goals and viewing each day's progress with optimism, exercising regularly for at least 30 minutes per day, and taking care of one's body by eating healthy and getting enough sleep.

Occasionally, over-the-counter medications may be used to alleviate stress symptoms, such as aspirin or ibuprofen for headaches, or antacids or antidiarrhea medications for upset stomachs. Alternative therapies may also be used, such as acupuncture, yoga, or relaxation methods.

Often, individuals may require a combination of treatment methods to prevent and maintain their stress. Additionally, individuals may have to try various coping methods before finding what works for them and fits in to their daily schedules.

DATA AND ANALYSES

Data

Table 43.1 Consequences of Unhealthy Sleeping Habits Based on Generation: United States, 2013

Generation	Age range	Feel sluggish or lazy	Difficulty concentrating or completing tasks	Unmotivated to take care of responsibilities
Millenial	18–33	60%	38%	34%
Generation X	34–47	58%	32%	23%
Baby Boomer	48–66	50%	27%	22%
Mature	67 and older	37%	11%	14%

Source: American Psychological Association. 2014. "Stress in America." Retrieved from: http://www.apa.org/news/press/releases/stress/2013/stress-report.pdf

Analysis

Table 43.1 presents the consequences of unhealthy sleeping habits based on generations in the United States. On average, younger generations, including Millenials and Generation X-ers, report getting fewer hours of sleep per night, as well as a lack of good-quality sleep. Twenty-nine percent of Millenials and 23% of Generation X-ers report that their sleep habits cause them stress, compared to 19% percent of Baby Boomers and only 7% of Matures. Generation X-ers report the fewest hours of sleep out of all groups; however, Millenials report poorer sleeping habits than all other groups. Due to these factors, both generations present a large gap between how well they are sleeping and how important sleep is to them.

Poor sleeping habits among younger generations present greater levels of stress and its negative symptoms. As the data shows, Millenials present the most feelings of sluggishness or laziness, difficulty concentrating or completing tasks, and lack of motivation to take care of responsibilities. Similarly, Generation X-ers present high levels of stress symptoms that stem from poor sleeping habits, followed by Baby Boomers and Matures.

Further research can examine why younger generations are experiencing poorer sleep habits and more negative stress symptoms compared to older generations, as well as determine how to improve sleep habits and decrease negative symptoms.

Data

Table 43.2 Stress Management Techniques of Teens vs. Adults: United States, 2013

Stress management technique	Percentage of teens	Percentage of adults
Play video games	46%	21%
Surf the Internet/Go online	43%	42%
Exercise or walk	37%	43%
Watch television or movies for over 2 hours per day	36%	40%
Play sports	28%	9%

Source: American Psychological Association. 2014. "Stress in America." Retrieved from: http://www.apa.org/news/press/releases/stress/2013/stress-report.pdf

Analysis

Table 43.2 presents stress management techniques in teens versus adults. The data shows that teens tend to seek more sedentary stress management techniques. Only 37% of teens exercise and 28% play sports to deal with stress, compared to 46% that play video games, 43% that go online, and 36% that watch television or movies.

It is important to observe and address stress management techniques, since teens who exercise report lower average stress levels. Additionally, teens who present a normal body mass index (BMI) also report lower stress levels than teens that are overweight or obese. Yet, there is a correlation between high stress levels and sedentary management techniques. For example, over half of teens with high stress levels say that they go online to manage their stress, while only 24% of teens with low stress go online. Similarly, 48% of teens with high stress watch television or movies to manage their stress, while only 20% of teens with low stress do the same.

By examining adults, it is apparent that although the most used stress management technique is exercising, they present high levels of sedentary management techniques as well. Additionally, adults are similar to teens in the fact that those who engage in physical activity for stress management report lower overall stress levels. Also, adults with higher stress levels tend to use sedentary stress management techniques. For example, only about one-third of adults who engage in sedentary management techniques report that they are effective in reducing stress levels, while about two-thirds who engage in physical activity report that their stress levels are reduced.

DISCUSSION QUESTIONS

1. Why do younger generations present poorer sleeping habits and more negative stress symptoms? How can their sleep habits be improved?
2. What other factors relate to negative stress symptoms in younger generations? How can these factors be addressed to reduce symptoms?
3. Why don't more teens and adults engage in physical activity as stress management techniques? How can more people become aware of the benefits of exercise and its effect on reducing stress levels?
4. Is there a correlation between teen and adult stress management techniques? For example, if more adults start using physical activity to deal with stress, will more teens engage in these activities as well?
5. Why do individuals with higher stress levels choose sedentary stress management techniques, even though these methods are not as effective?

44

STROKE

INTRODUCTION

Understanding Stroke

In 2010, cerebrovascular diseases were the fourth leading cause of death in the United States after heart disease, cancer, and chronic lower respiratory diseases. This complex health issue refers to any condition that affects the unaffected flowing of blood to and from the brain. The most common form of cerebrovascular disease is stroke, which damages brain cells when blood supply to them is interrupted or floods the areas between them.

There are two major types of stroke, including ischemic and hemorrhagic strokes. While the more frequent ischemic strokes involve blocked arteries, hemorrhagic strokes deal with ruptured arteries. There are also subcategories of these strokes, like the transient ischemic attack mini-stroke, intracerebral hemorrhage stroke, and subarachnoid hemorrhage stroke. In many cases, the severity of these strokes allows them to have the potential to kill or leave a person with a serious long-term disability.

Signs

Most of the signs that indicate an individual is having a stroke happen immediately and seemingly without cause. However, they are a direct result of at least one of the major types of stroke. Affecting different parts of the body, these signs include very sudden:

- Numbness in the face, arms, or legs
- Weakness in the face, arms, or legs
- Confusion
- Trouble talking or forming words
- Trouble understanding speech
- Difficulty seeing
- Difficulty walking
- Loss of balance
- Lack of coordination
- Sharp, pounding headache

Most signs of stroke, like numbness or weakness of the face, arms, or legs, usually concentrate on one of these three areas or occur on only one side of the individual's body. This is because one side of the brain affects the opposite side of the body. For example, if a person has a stroke on the left half of their brain, the right side of their body will experience one or a combination of the aforementioned signs.

With transient ischemic strokes in particular, symptoms occur suddenly and fade away after several minutes. Although these signs may seem temporary or inconsequential, they are extremely damaging in the long term and require immediate attention as they are likely to reappear.

Risk Factors

There are several factors and lifestyle choices that put individuals at risk for stroke. These include:

- Obesity
- High cholesterol
- High blood pressure
- Heart palpitations
- Smoking
- Diabetes
- Previous strokes

While some of these factors may not be completely controlled, many of them can be managed to prevent an occurrence or reoccurrence of stroke. Usually, consistent physical activity and a healthy diet will help to offset them.

Treatment

There are various stages of treatment for people who experience a stroke, starting from the moment symptoms occur. Since this cerebrovascular condition is an emergency that puts the survival of brain function at stake, it requires immediate medical attention. After getting to a hospital, patients are normally given brain scans not only to diagnose the stroke type but also give medical professionals a chance to see where exactly it occurred in the brain so that they can begin to efficiently work to fix it.

A thrombolytic drug like tissue plasminogen activator may be administered to a patient suffering from an ischemic stroke. This medicine is crucial in quickly removing blood clots cause by this type of stroke, and has been found to increase the probability of major disability after a full recovery.

For ischemic and hemorrhagic stroke patients, an endovascular procedure can be performed. This involves catheters, or long tubes, that are inserted through the patient's arm or leg arteries. Once the tubes are led through the body and reach the obstruction in the brain, doctors can remove a clot or install mechanical coils to prevent any further ruptures.

The last option is surgery. Exclusively for hemorrhagic patients who are experiencing major bleeding, surgery allows medical professionals to stop and fasten the stroke-affected area with devices like metal clips. Because this treatment deals with the delicate areas of the brain, it is undoubtedly the most dangerous—albeit life-saving—option.

However, stroke treatment does not stop with getting to a hospital, taking medicine, or undergoing surgery. A majority of individuals must take on rehabilitation, including speech therapy, physical therapy, occupational therapy, and psychological therapy, to fully recover after these events. Participating in rehabilitation sessions allows those affected by stroke to relearn any activities like talking, walking, eating, or writing that they might have lost the ability to do or to remember how to do, as well as to continue on their path toward their life before the stroke.

DATA AND ANALYSES

Data

Table 44.1 Percentage of Stroke Hospitalization and Characteristics in the United States, 1989, 1999, and 2009

Characteristic	1989	1999	2009
Total stroke hospitalizations	795,000	961,000	971,000
Average age of hospital inpatients (years)	71	71	70
	Percentage		
Proportion by sex			
Male	43	45	48
Female	57	55	52
Proportion by age group			
Under 65 years	24	27	34
65 years and older	76	73	66
Proportions with comorbidities			
Diabetes	18	23	23
Atrial fibrillation	10	12	12
At least one of the above comorbidities	65	91	94
Hypertension	37	55	58

Source: http://www.cdc.gov/nchs/data/databriefs/db95.htm

Analysis

There have been several changes in the amount of stroke hospitalizations and the characteristics, like sex, that defined them from 1989 to 2009. Table 44.1 shows that hospitalizations jumped from 795,000 in 1989 to almost a million in 1999 and 2009. Of these hospitalizations, there were generally more female patients than male ones for all three years, but the gap between the two sexes narrowed by 2009 with male percentages increasing and female percentages decreasing over time.

The average age of stroke patients, around 70–71 years, remained the same throughout the 20-year time frame. However, the number of patients aged 65 years and older decreased by 10% in 2009, and those aged 65 years and younger increased by 10% by 2009.

Interestingly, a majority of stroke victims also suffered from diabetes, hypertension, or atrial fibrillation before or at the time of their hospitalization. The number of patients hospitalized with one or more of these comorbidities increased into the new century. Those with hypertension in particular more than doubled from 1989 to 2009.

Data

Table 44.2 Percentage of Stroke Prevalence in the United States Among Various Races and Ethnicities, 2006–2010

	2006	2007	2008	2009	2010
White	2.4%	2.4%	2.3%	2.2%	2.4%
Black	3.7%	4.1%	4.1%	3.7%	3.9%
Hispanic	2.5%	2.9%	2.7%	2.6%	2.5%
Asian, Native Hawaiian, or other Pacific Islander	2.3%	1.5%	1.6%	1.5%	1.5%
American Indian or Alaska Native	5.5%	5.3%	5.6%	4.4%	5.9%

Source: http://www.cdc.gov/mmwr/preview/mmwrhtml/mm6120a5.htm?s_cid=mm6120a5_w

Analysis

Table 44.2 shows the correlation between stroke and race or ethnicity between 2006 and 2010. Between these years, American Indians and Alaska Natives consistently exhibited the majority of stroke incidences out of all other races and ethnicities, followed by black men and women, whose percentages were more than double those of whites, Hispanics, Asians, Native Hawaiian, and other Pacific Islanders.

Asians, Native Hawaiians, and other Pacific Islanders composed the only group to show a decrease in stroke occurrence during this time frame, starting with 2.3% in 2006 and remaining between 1.5% and 1.6% just one year later and into 2010. Hispanics showed no change at all from 2006 to 2010.

DISCUSSION QUESTIONS

1. The word "cerebrovascular" is derived from "cerebro," which refers to the brain, and "vascular," which denotes blood vessels like the arteries and veins. As a member of this disease category, how does a stroke fit into this etymology of cerebrovascular?
2. What risk factors or lifestyle factors might cause American Indians and Native Alaskans to be particularly prone to strokes, as shown in Table 44.2?
3. At the hospital, patients must take brain scans to diagnose a stroke. What other conditions or diseases might doctors mistake a stroke as, judging from symptoms alone?

4. Surgery is recommended almost exclusively for hemorrhagic stroke patients. Why might surgery not be the most effective option for victims of ischemic stroke?

5. Although strokes are a leading cause of death in the United States, many people are not aware of it and cannot even identify sign and symptoms. What type of programs can be created to inform others about this disease?

45

SUICIDE

INTRODUCTION

Understanding Suicide

Suicide is one of the most significant public health problems that has affected people for centuries and continues to affect people around the world today. Unlike most illness or disease, it does not have a cure and is caused deliberately by the person themselves.

Suicide is when a person ends his or her life. A suicide attempt is when a person is unsuccessful in killing him- or herself. There are several different methods that people use to commit suicide. Some of the most common methods involve:

- Firearm
- Poison
- Suffocation
- Hanging
- Exsanguination (loss of blood)
- Drowning
- Drug or alcohol overdose
- Jumping from a height

Suicide has several different names, but is most commonly referred to as intentional self-harm or self-inflicted injury by medical professionals. It is worth noting that suicide is different from accidents. While suicide is intentional, accidents are unintentional.

Risk Factors

Although suicide is not a "traditional" illness or disease, and does not have one single cause, there are still several risk factors involved with it. The main risk factors that make a person more likely to attempt suicide—but that do not necessarily guarantee the occurrence and completion of suicide—include but are not limited to:

- Previous suicide attempts
- History of depression
- History of mental illness
- Family history of suicide or violence
- Alcohol or drug abuse
- Physical illness
- Feelings of alienation

Effects

It is typically difficult for people who survive suicide attempts to return to their daily lives and carry them out normally. Many times, they are forced to experience short- and long-term effects that act as reminders of their failed suicidal act and further diminish their perceived quality of life. These effects can sometimes lead to another suicide attempt if the person does not seek help. Some short-term and long-term effects of suicide include:

- Broken bones
- Organ failure
- Brain damage
- Scarring
- Weakness and numbness in affected areas
- Injured tendons, nerves, vessels, and muscles
- Declining physical health
- Social isolation
- Depression
- Declining mental health

It is important to understand that suicide does not solely affect the person who commits or attempts the act. Whether someone successfully ends their life or fails trying to do so, their family members and friends who care for them can be impacted negatively. More often than not, these impacts are emotional or mental rather than physical. Keeping this in mind, it is not uncommon for loved ones of the suicide or suicide-attempt victim to experience bouts of depression, confusion, anger, shame, guilt, and shock.

DATA AND ANALYSES

Data

Table 45.1 Death Rates for the 15 Leading Causes of Death in the United States, Age-adjusted, 2010 and 2011

Cause of death	2010 death rate	2011 death rate
1. Diseases of heart	179.1	173.7
2. Malignant neoplasms	172.8	168.6
3. Chronic lower respiratory diseases	42.2	42.7
4. Cerebrovascular diseases	39.1	37.9
5. Accidents (unintentional injuries)	38.0	38.0
6. Alzheimer's disease	25.1	24.6
7. Diabetes mellitus	20.8	21.5
8. Influenza and pneumonia	15.1	15.7
9. Nephritis, nephrotic syndrome, and nephrosis	15.3	13.4
10. Intentional self-harm (suicide)	**12.1**	**12.0**
11. Septicemia	10.6	10.5
12. Chronic liver disease and cirrhosis	9.4	9.7
13. Essential hypertension and hypertensive renal disease	8.0	8.0
14. Parkinson's disease	6.8	7.0
15. Pneumonitis due to solids and liquids	5.1	5.3

Note: Rates are per 100,000 population.

Source: http://www.cdc.gov/nchs/data/nvsr/nvsr61/nvsr61_06.pdf

Analysis

Table 45.1 provides an overview of the 15 leading causes of death in the United States in 2010 and 2011, along with their corresponding age-adjusted death rates. Of these 15 causes of death, intentional self-harm and suicide had the tenth highest death rate during both years. The death rate for suicide was virtually the same in 2010 and

2011. With the 12.0 in 2010 and 12.1 in 2011, there was only a −0.8% change. Although the suicide death rates are small compared to other causes of death higher up on the table, the fact that intentional self-harm sits among fatal diseases and illnesses that cannot be controlled shows just how significant this public health problem is.

Data

Table 45.2 Number of Suicides in the United States Among Persons Aged 35 to 64 Years, 1999 and 2010

	1999	2010
35–39 years old	3,286	3,084
40–44 years old	3,180	3,487
45–49 years old	2,817	4,372
50–54 years old	2,264	4,427
55–59 years old	1,678	3,760
60–64 years old	1,218	2,624
Total	14,443	21,754

Source: http://www.cdc.gov/mmwr/preview/mmwrhtml/mm6217a1.htm?s_cid=mm6217a1_w

Analysis

Table 45.2 shows the number of suicides by age group (ages 35–64) in the United States in the years 1999 and 2010. In every age group—except for the 35–39 age group—there was an increase in the number of suicides. In some cases, the numbers almost doubled. For example, with the 55–59 age range, the numbers jumped from 1,678 suicides in 1999 to 3,760 suicides in 2010. Taking into account all age groups, there were 14,443 total suicides in 1999 and 21,754 total suicides in 2010.

Data

Table 45.3 Percentage of U.S. High School Students Considering, Planning, or Attempting Suicide, by Sex, 2009

Males	Percentage
Considered	10.5%
Planned	8.6%
Attempted	4.6%

Females	Percentage
Considered	17.4%
Planned	13.2%
Attempted	8.1%

Note: Data takes into account reports in the past 12 months, at time of survey.

Source: http://www.cdc.gov/violenceprevention/suicide/statistics/youth_risk.html

Analysis

Table 45.3 demonstrates the percentage of male and female high school students in the United States who considered, planned, or attempted suicide in 2009, within 12 months of the survey being given. In general, more female students considered, planned, and attempted suicide than male students. In fact, the female data is almost double that of the male data in all three categories taken into account by the study. While 17.4% of female students *considered* suicide, 10.5% of male students did. While 13.2% female students *planned* suicide, 8.6% of male students did. Finally, while 8.1% of female student *attempted* suicide, 4.6% of male students did.

Interestingly, studies by the Centers for Disease Control and Prevention have shown that women *are* more likely to have suicidal thoughts than men, which supplements the data shown in Table 45.3. Although men are less likely to have suicidal thoughts, they are four times more likely to die from suicide than women if they attempt it.

DISCUSSION QUESTIONS

1. Suicide attempts are far more common among young adults under 30 than they are among adults over 30. Considering broad and more detailed aspects, what might make the former age group struggle with suicide more than the latter age group?
2. According to the data above, more female high school students consider, plan, and attempt suicide than male high school students. What are some possible physical or emotional reasons for this discrepancy between genders?
3. Suicide continues to be one of the ten leading causes of death in the United States. What measures can be taken—and taken by whom—to raise awareness for this public health problem in an effort to reduce the death rate?

4. Unlike other illnesses, diseases, and conditions, suicide does not have a traditional "cure" and is caused deliberately. For what other reasons is suicide different from health issues like cancer, hypertension, and heart disease?

5. The total number of suicides for almost every age group in the United States increased significantly from 1999 to 2010. What are some possible reasons for this jump, and how do you think the numbers will compare in the next ten years?

46

TEENAGE PREGNANCY

INTRODUCTION

Understanding Teenage Pregnancy

A pregnancy is considered an adolescent or teenage pregnancy when the female is younger than 20 years old. Adolescent females can become pregnant if they have vaginal sex with a male any time after the start of regular monthly periods, which typically occurs around age 12 or 13. Teenage pregnancies carry extra health risks to both the mother and the baby, as any pregnancy under the age of 20 poses more danger than pregnancy in older females. Fortunately, teenage pregnancies have been declining in the United States due to an increased use and availability of contraceptives.

Symptoms

The earliest symptoms of pregnancy appear within the first few weeks after conception. Some symptoms could indicate that an individual is getting sick or getting their period; however, missing a period is the biggest indication that a female may be pregnant. All females experience different symptoms during their pregnancy, but common early symptoms of pregnancy that occur during the first trimester (weeks 1–12) include:

- Tender, swollen breasts caused by hormonal changes. Breasts may also feel fuller and heavier.

- Nausea with or without vomiting, also known as morning sickness. Morning sickness can occur at any time of the day or night and may be heightened by certain smells.
- Increased urination
- Fatigue, caused by an increase in progesterone levels
- Food cravings or aversions, caused by hormonal changes
- Spotting or vaginal bleeding that is much lighter than a normal period and occurs about 10–14 days after conception
- Cramping
- Mood swings
- Dizziness, caused by dilation of blood vessels and a drop in blood pressure
- Constipation, caused by the slowing of the digestive system that results from hormonal changes
- Weight change

While some symptoms will fade by the second trimester (weeks 13–28), other bodily changes will become more noticeable. Certain changes include: body aches, stretch marks, darkening of the skin around nipples, numb or tingling hands, itching on the abdomen and soles of the feet, and swelling of the ankles, fingers, and face.

During the third trimester (weeks 29–40), females tend to experience shortness of breath and have to urinate frequently as the baby grows and puts more pressure on the organs. In addition, females can experience heartburn, hemorrhoids, trouble sleeping, contractions, and continued swelling of the ankles, fingers, and face.

Risk Factors

Risk factors for teenage pregnancy include individual and environmental factors. Individual risk factors such as drug and alcohol use, lack of knowledge about sex or contraception, lack of goals, low self-esteem, being a victim of sexual abuse, poor school performance, having sex at a young age, and already having a baby all contribute to an increased risk of teenage pregnancy. Additionally, social factors such as pressure to have sex, dating at an early age, dating older men, and having friends that are sexually active contribute to increased risk of teen pregnancy, as well as family factors including poor parental supervision, limited or negative family interaction, single-parent families, and family history of teenage pregnancy.

While it is important to be aware of the risk factors for teenage pregnancy, it is also important to understand that teenage pregnancy is a major risk factor for other medical conditions. Teenage pregnancies put mothers at a higher risk of developing medical complications, such as: preeclampsia, also known as high blood pressure, which can harm the kidneys or even be fatal; anemia, which can lead to fatigue and affect the baby's development; toxemia, which can put the mother in a coma; and placenta previa, which can cause life-threatening bleeding. Teen pregnancies also put the baby at higher risk of developing conditions such as premature birth and low birth weight, both of which can affect development of the baby and result in lifelong complications.

Diagnosis

Teens may notice a missed period or suspect that they are pregnant due to apparent symptoms. Pelvic examinations may be used to reveal bluish or purple coloring of the vaginal walls and cervix, as well as the softening and enlargement of the uterus, all of which indicate pregnancy. Blood or urine pregnancy tests and pregnancy ultrasounds should also be administered to confirm pregnancy.

Pregnancy tests work by detecting the hormone human chorionic gonadotropin (hCG), which is only present in the urine or blood when a female is pregnant, as it is produced when a fertilized eggs implants in the uterus. The pregnancy hormone hCG is normally produced about six days after conception, but may not occur until after the first missed period; therefore, results will be more accurate the longer an individual waits. The amount of hCG also increases each day after implantation.

While blood tests can detect hCG more quickly, many females use home pregnancy tests to initially determine if they are pregnant. Home pregnancy tests will be most accurate if used a week after a missed period. Home pregnancy tests are inexpensive, easy to use, and can be found at most supermarkets or drug stores. However, when using a home pregnancy test, it is important to repeat the test a few days later or confirm results with a medical professional, as the home pregnancy test may be faulty or unable to detect the pregnancy hormone hCG if used too early.

Medical Support and Treatment

A pregnant teen has various options, which include raising the baby with support, adoption, and, in some cases, abortion. Decisions on how to deal with the pregnancy should be considered very carefully, as there are different methods, benefits, and risks for each option. If the teen chooses to continue the pregnancy, early prenatal care should be administered in order to reduce medical complications for the mother and the baby. During pregnancy, teens should be educated to stop smoking, drinking alcohol, and using drugs. Additionally, pregnant teens should make routine check-ups with a doctor to monitor their health, as well as the baby's health. Pregnant teens should also be tested for sexually transmitted diseases if they have not been already. Pregnant teens should be aware of proper nutrition, as they require more folic acid, calcium, iron, protein, and other nutrients that can be supplemented with vitamins. Additionally, regular exercise can help prepare for labor and maintain health. Childbirth classes and educating oneself about pregnancy will also help ensure a healthy pregnancy, as additional factors such as sleep, gaining weight, preparing for labor, and establishing post-pregnancy plans are important to consider. Teenagers carrying out their pregnancy should ask for support, as the pregnancy will cause emotional, physical, and environmental changes.

A reduction in teenage pregnancies and related medical complications that occur for the mother and baby can be prevented by six objectives outlined by the World Health Organization: reducing marriages before the age of 18, reducing pregnancies before the age of 20, increasing contraceptive use by adolescents, reducing sex among adolescents, reducing unsafe abortions among adolescents, and increasing prenatal and postnatal care among adolescents.

DATA AND ANALYSES

Data

Table 46.1 Never-married Females Aged 15–19 Who Have Ever Had Sexual Intercourse by Race/ethnicity: United States, 1988–2010

Race/ethnicity	Percentage in year 1988	Percentage in year 1995	Percentage in year 2002	Percentage in years 2006–2010
Hispanic	45.8%	52.7%	37.4%	42.1%
Non-Hispanic white	50.4%	48.5%	45.1%	41.9%
Non-Hispanic black	60.4%	59.3%	56.9%	46.4%
All races	51.1%	49.3%	45.5%	42.6%

Source: Centers for Disease Control and Prevention. 2011. "Teenagers in the United States: Sexual activity, contraceptive use, and childbearing, 2006–2010." Retrieved from: http://www.cdc.gov/nchs/data/series/sr_23/sr23_031.pdf

Analysis

Table 46.1 presents that about 43% of never-married teenage females have had sexual intercourse at least once during the years of 2006 through 2010, which is a substantial decrease from the estimated 51% of sexually active teenagers in 1988. The data presents a steady decline in teenage sexual activity throughout the 1988–2010 period. The most significant decrease from recent years was presented in non-Hispanic black females, as an estimated 57% of sexually active females dropped to about 46% from 2002 to the 2006–2010 period. Generally, non-Hispanic black females presented the highest rates of teenage sexual activity; however, Hispanic rates have fluctuated over the years. Further research can examine the cause of the fluctuation in Hispanic teenagers and how sexual intercourse rates relate to teenage pregnancy rates.

Data

Table 46.2 Use of Contraception at First Sex Among Females Aged 15–19 by Race/ethnicity: United States, 2002 vs. 2006–2010

Race/ethnicity	Percentage of use in year 2002	Percentage of use in years 2006–2010
Hispanic	66%	74%
Non-Hispanic white	78%	82%
Non-Hispanic black	71%	71%
All races	74.5%	78%

Source: Centers for Disease Control and Prevention. 2011. "Teenagers in the United States: Sexual activity, contraceptive use, and childbearing, 2006–2010." Retrieved from: http://www.cdc.gov/nchs/data/series/sr_23/sr23_031.pdf

Analysis

Table 46.2 presents the use of contraception by race/ethnicity in teenagers who have sexual intercourse for the first time. During the 2006–2010 year period, about 78% of females used a contraceptive method, which is a slight increase from the estimated 74.5% of contraceptive users in 2002. Further data elaborated to present the condom as the most common method of contraception at first intercourse, accounting for 68% of contraceptive methods. The pill, or birth control, was the second most common method of contraception at first intercourse, accounting for 16% of contraceptive methods.

Contraceptive use at first intercourse was highest among non-Hispanic white females. Non-Hispanic black females presented no change in contraceptive use from 2002 to the 2006–2010 period, while Hispanics dramatically increased the amount of contraceptive use by 8%. Further research can determine even more ways to increase the awareness and availability of contraception for all teenagers so that teenage pregnancy rates can continue to be reduced.

Data

Table 46.3 Birth Rates per 1,000 Females Aged 15–19 Years Old by Race/ethnicity: United States, 2009–2011

Race/ethnicity	2009 birth rates	2010 birth rates	2011 birth rates
Asian/Pacific Islander	13	11	10
Non-Hispanic white	26	24	22
American Indian/Alaska Native	44	39	36
Non-Hispanic black	57	52	47
Hispanic	64	56	49
Average for all races/ethnicities	38	34	31

Source: Centers for Disease Control and Prevention. 2011. "Teen pregnancy." Retrieved from: http://www.cdc.gov/teenpregnancy/aboutteenpreg.htm

Analysis

In 2011, 31.3 per 1,000 females aged 15–19 experienced a live birth, resulting in a total of 329,797 babies. Table 46.3 presents a steady decrease in teenage pregnancies from 2009 to 2011. Broken up by race/ethnicity, all groups presented a decline in teenage pregnancies during this time period. The greatest decrease was seen in Hispanic females, whose birth rates decreased 15% from 2009 to 2011. However, Hispanics also account for the most live births in the United States. Combined with non-Hispanic blacks, these two groups accounted for 57% of teenage pregnancies during 2011. Asian/Pacific Islanders presented the lowest teenage pregnancy rates, followed by non-Hispanic whites. Further research can examine what socioeconomic factors play a role in teenage pregnancy rates and help explain why the rates differ among different races/ethnicities.

DISCUSSION QUESTIONS

1. How do sexual activity and teenage pregnancy rates in the United States relate to rates in other nations? If rates are lower in other nations, what can be learned or implemented to reduce United States teenage pregnancy rates even further?
2. Why are teenage sexual intercourse rates higher for non-Hispanic blacks in the United States? How does data collection methods affect the results?
3. What accounts for the decrease in teenage sexual intercourse over the 1988–2010 period? How can these rates continue to be reduced?
4. Why have Hispanic rates of teenage sexual intercourse fluctuated over the years? How can these rates be maintained and reduced?
5. Why do you think that contraceptive use is comparatively low among the Hispanic population? How can contraceptive use among the Hispanic population, as well as all sexually active teenagers, be increased?
6. How do rates of contraception at first sexual intercourse relate to continued contraceptive use?

47

THYROID CANCER

INTRODUCTION

Understanding Thyroid Cancer

Thyroid cancer originates in the thyroid gland, which is located below the Adam's apple in the front of the neck. Two lobes are connected by an isthmus to make up the thyroid gland. Within the thyroid gland is two central types of cells: follicular cells, which use iodine from the blood to make thyroid hormones that regulate metabolism; and parafollicular cells, also known as C cells, which make calcitonin hormones that regulate how the body uses calcium. Lymphocytes and stromal cells are also found in the thyroid gland. The severity of cancer depends on which cell the cancer originates from.

Differentiated thyroid cancers, which develop from follicular cells, include papillary carcinomas, follicular carcinomas, and Hurthle cell carcinomas. Papillary carcinomas account for the majority of differentiated thyroid cancers. This type of cancer usually develops slowly, only in one lobe of the thyroid gland. The subtypes of papillary carcinomas include: the follicular subtype, which is the most common and has a good prognosis; and columnar, tall cell, insular, and diffuse sclerosing subtypes, which tend to progress more quickly. Follicular carcinomas typically spread to the lungs or bones. Hurthle cell carcinomas, also known as oxyphil cell carcinomas, are harder to find and treat.

More rare types of thyroid cancer include: medullary thyroid carcinoma (MTC), anaplastic carcinoma, and thyroid lymphoma. Medullary thyroid carcinomas develops from C cells, often releasing excess calcitonin and carcinoembryonic antigen protein. Subtypes of MTC include: sporadic MTC, which accounts for the majority of MTC cases and only affects one lobe; and familial MTC, which is inherited and develops at an early age, affecting both lobes. Anaplastic carcinomas develop from existing papillary or follicular cancers, often called undifferentiated carcinomas because the cancer cells appear very different than regular thyroid cells. Thyroid lymphoma that develops from lymphocytes and thyroid sarcomas that develop from stromal cells are extremely rare. Parathyroid cancers are also extremely rare, affecting the four small glands attached to the back of the thyroid gland.

SYMPTOMS

Some individuals may not present any symptoms, and the tumor will only be detected during a routine physical exam completed by their doctor; however, thyroid cancers can produce any of these symptoms:

- Lumps in the neck that may or may not grow quickly
- Swelling in the neck
- Pain in the front of the neck that may extend to the ears
- Hoarseness or other permanent voice changes
- Difficulty swallowing
- Difficulty breathing
- Constant coughing unrelated to a common cold

Many of these symptoms can also be caused by other cancers or noncancerous conditions, so it is important to see a medical professional if any of the symptoms are present.

Risk Factors

Multiple risk factors affect an individual's chance of developing thyroid cancer, including:

- Gender: Females are more likely than males to develop thyroid cancer.
- Age: Females aged 40–50 are at the highest risk of developing thyroid cancers, while males aged 60–70 are at the highest risk.

- Diet: Diets that lack iodine increase the risk of follicular thyroid cancers, as well as papillary cancer if the person is also exposed to radioactivity.
- Radiation: Medical treatments and fallout from power plant accidents or nuclear weapons are directly related to increases in thyroid cancer. The larger amount of exposure, the greater the risk of developing thyroid cancer.
- Family/past medical history: Most individuals who develop thyroid cancer do not have an inherited condition or family history of thyroid cancer; however, the presence of thyroid cancer in a relative does increase the risk of development. Also, specific conditions have been linked to an increased risk of thyroid cancer. For example, about 1 in 3 medullary thyroid carcinomas are caused by inheriting an abnormal gene called RET. Additionally, familial adenomatous poluposis, cowden disease, carney complex, and familial nonmedullary thyroid carcinoma all increase the risk of developing thyroid cancer.

Diagnosis

Enlargement of the thyroid gland is common and can be detected by a doctor. Often, the cause of the enlargement, or goiter, is caused by an imbalance of hormones and does not present cancer; however, about 1 in 20 nodules or lumps in the thyroid gland are cancerous. Many thyroid cancers can be detected early, leading to more successful treatment. Blood tests and thyroid ultrasounds can be used to detect changes or enlargements in the thyroid; however, these screening tests are not recommended unless an individual presents risk factors of developing thyroid cancer.

The actual diagnosis of thyroid cancer is conducted with a physical examination, imaging tests, blood tests, and, most importantly, a biopsy. Ultrasounds are the most commonly used imaging tests, as they can determine if a thyroid nodule is solid or filled with fluid. Solid nodules are typically more cancerous. The number and the size of the thyroid nodules can also be determined, as well as the enlargement of nearby lymph nodes, which indicate the spread of thyroid cancer. Another way of determining whether the thyroid cancer has spread is radioiodine scans. To conduct this test, a small amount of radioactive iodine is swallowed in pill form or injected into a vein and absorbed by the thyroid gland, allowing a thyroid scan to measure the amount of radiation concentrated in the gland. Abnormal cells will have less or more radioactivity than surrounding tissue. Similarly, positron emission tomography (PET) scans may be used in cases where radioactive iodine cannot be used, such as with MTC cells that do not absorb iodine. PET scans inject a radioactive sugar substance, known as FDG, into the blood that is then absorbed by the thyroid gland. Additionally, computed tomography (CT) scans and magnetic resonance imaging (MRI) scans can also determine the location and size of the thyroid cancer and whether it has spread, but are used less frequently.

Blood tests can be used to determine whether the thyroid is functioning normally. Blood tests will typically examine: thyroid-stimulating hormone (TSH), which is high if the thyroid is not making enough hormones and can help determine which imaging tests to use; T3 and T4 thyroid hormones; thyroglobulin, which can detect existing thyroid cancer cells after surgery; calcitonin, which is high in individuals with MTC; and carcinoembryonic antigen (CEA), which also helps diagnose MTC.

Ultimately, a biopsy is needed to diagnose thyroid cancer. A biopsy removes cells from the thyroid gland and examines them under a microscope to look for abnormalities. Typically, a fine needle aspiration is used, which can be performed in a doctor's office by placing a thin needle directly in to the lump or nodule. Biopsies are typically conducted on all thyroid nodules or lumps that are about a half-inch across, meaning they are large enough to be felt. An ultrasound may accompany the doctor during the biopsy, especially when sampling smaller nodules. If diagnosis is still not clear after a fine needle aspiration biopsy, other procedures may be used to resample the cells, such as: core biopsy, surgical biopsy, or lobectomy, which is removal of half of the thyroid gland.

Treatment

The stage of thyroid cancer is one of the most important factors in determining treatment. The most common system used to stage thyroid cancer was developed by the American Joint Committee on Cancer, known as the TNM system: T indicates the size of the tumor and whether it has spread; N describes the extent that the cancer has spread, specifically examining the lymph nodes; and M determines whether the cancer has spread to other organs in the body, most commonly the lungs, liver and bones. The numbers 0–4 are stated after the TNM categorization to indicate the severity of the cancer. The stage is then determined by grouping the TNM categorization and the subsequent level of severity, resulting in stages I–IV.

Differentiated thyroid cancers and MTC can appear at any stage, while anaplastic thyroid cancer is always considered stage IV. Fortunately, most cases of thyroid cancer can be cured with treatment.

Surgery is very common in treating thyroid cancer, as removal of the entire thyroid or thyroidectomy is often used to reduce chances of recurrence. Enlarged lymph nodes that present cancerous symptoms may also be removed during surgery. Occasionally, only a portion of the thyroid will be removed, which is known as a thyroid lobectomy. Following surgery, thyroid hormone medications must be taken for life in order to supply the missing hormones regularly produced by the thyroid gland and suppress the production of TSH from the pituitary gland as high TSH levels can cause the cancer to recur.

Additional treatment that follows surgery includes radioactive iodine therapy, which removes any cancerous cells that were left over from surgery. If the cancer continues to grow even after these methods, external radiation therapy may be used to slow the spread of cancer. External radiation therapy, which aims high-energy beams at precise points on the body, can also be used for individuals that cannot undergo surgery. Other options for thyroid cancer that cannot be cured with surgery include: chemotherapy, which is a drug treatment that kills cancer cells; alcohol ablation, which injects alcohol in to the cancerous cells via ultrasound; and targeted drug therapy, which uses medications to attack the cancerous cells.

DATA AND ANALYSES

Data

Table 47.1 Percent of New Cases of Thyroid Cancer and Related Deaths by Age Group: United States, 2007–2011 and 2006–2010

Age group	Percent of new cases, 2007–2011	Percent of deaths, 2006–2010
0–20 years	1.8%	0.1%
20–34 years	15.1%	0.9%
35–44 years	19.6%	2.4%
45–54 years	24.2%	8.0%
55–64 years	19.9%	16.9%
65–74 years	12.3%	24.7%
75–84 years	5.7%	29.5%
>84 years	1.4%	17.6%

Source: National Cancer Institute. 2011. "Surveillance, epidemiology, and end results program." Retrieved from: http://seer.cancer.gov/statfacts/html/thyro.html

Analysis

Table 47.1 presents the percentage of new cases of thyroid cancer from 2007 through 2011 and the percentage of deaths from thyroid cancer from 2006 through 2010 by age group. Results show that the number of new cases of thyroid cancer was 12.9 per 100,000 males and females per year. The number of deaths was 0.5 per 100,000 males and females per year. Broken down by age, the data presents that the median age at diagnosis is 50 years old, and the median age at death is 73 years old.

Evidently, the percentage of new cases of thyroid cancer occur mostly between the ages of 45 and 54, followed by 55–64 years old and 35–44 years old. These results comply with the risk factors related to age, which state that women aged 40–50 are at the highest risk of developing thyroid cancer, while males develop it a few years later. As females present more thyroid cancer cases than males, the 50-year-old median age of diagnosis is supported.

Additionally, the data presents that death rates increase with age. The majority of deaths occur between the ages of 75 and 84 years of age, followed by 65–74 years of age. By examining the relationship between the median age of diagnosis and the median age of death, researchers can further examine the treatment methods used to extend survival rates among thyroid cancer patients.

Data

Table 47.2 Number of New Cases of Thyroid Cancer and Related Deaths per 100,000 Persons by Race/ethnicity and Sex: United States, 2007–2011 and 2006–2010

Race/ethnicity	New cases: females, 2007–2011	Deaths: females, 2006–2010	New cases: males, 2007–2011	Deaths: males, 2006–2010
All races	19.1	0.5	6.4	0.5
White	20.4	0.5	6.9	0.5
Black	11.3	0.6	3.3	0.4
Asian/Pacific Islander	18.5	0.9	5.7	0.5
American Indian/ Alaska Native	11.8	Not shown, <16 cases	3.4	Not shown, <16 cases
Hispanic	17.2	0.7	4.7	0.5
Non-Hispanic	19.7	0.5	6.8	0.5

Source: National Cancer Institute. 2011. "Surveillance, epidemiology, and end results program." Retrieved from: http://seer.cancer.gov/statfacts/html/thyro.html

Analysis

Table 47.2 examines the number of new cases of thyroid cancer and related deaths per 100,000 persons. Broken down by race/ethnicity and sex, various trends resulted. Evidently, females account for more than three times the amount of new cases of thyroid cancer than males; however, the death rates are equal for both genders. White individuals account for the most new cases of thyroid cancer, followed by non-Hispanics and Asian/Pacific Islanders. Interestingly, Asian/Pacific Islanders account for the most deaths related to thyroid cancer, followed by Hispanic females. All other race/ethnicities have similar death rates per 100,000 persons.

By examining the relationship between thyroid cancer prevalence and mortality among race/ethnicity, researchers can determine why Asian/Pacific Islanders are affected more by the disease than other races.

DISCUSSION QUESTIONS

1. What treatment methods are responsible for the gap between the median age of diagnosis of thyroid cancer and the median age of death? How can the survival rates be extended even further?
2. Why do the majority of thyroid cancer diagnoses occur between the ages of 45 and 54? What makes these ages a higher risk factor for developing thyroid cancer?
3. Why are Asian/Pacific Islanders affected the most by thyroid cancer?
4. Whites present the most new cases of thyroid cancer; however, they do not account for the most deaths related to thyroid cancer. What is the reasoning for this? Does access to certain treatment methods affect the prognoses of thyroid cancer?
5. How do the different types of cancer acquired relate to mortality rates? Also, which types of cancer are responsible for the most new cases?

48

VACCINES AND IMMUNIZATIONS

INTRODUCTION

Understanding Vaccines and Immunizations

The terms vaccine and immunization are interchangeable, refer-ring to the safe and effective injection of a small amount of a virus or bacteria that is weakened or killed to act as an imitation of the real disease. Before vaccines, the only way to acquire immunity against a disease was to contract the disease and survive it, known as naturally acquired immunity. With naturally acquired immunity, individuals suffer the symptoms, complications, and risks of the disease, which were often fatal. Natural acquired immunity also allowed for the spread of the diseases.

Vaccines now provide artificially acquired immunity, which prevent infection by triggering the body's immune response and prompting the production of antibodies that fight against the virus or bacteria that cause disease. This prepares the immune system for future interactions with the actual disease-causing virus or bac-teria, either fully preventing the disease from developing in the body or at least reducing its severity. According to the Centers for Disease Control and Prevention, vaccines are 90–100% effective.

Immunizations protect individuals from serious diseases and prevent the spread of the diseases to others, both major goals of public health. While some vaccines only need to be administered one time, others require updates for continuous protection.

Immunizations for Children

According to the World Health Organization, immunizations currently prevent an estimated two to three million deaths per year; however, 22.6 million infants across the globe still do not receive vaccinations. In the United States, proof of immunization is required for enrollment in many schools or daycares; therefore, it is important to understand which vaccines children require. Additionally, within the first year of life, newborns lose the immunity that they had built up in their mother's womb, increasing their susceptibility to disease. At a young age, a child's immune system may not be strong enough to fight the disease, leading to fatalities. Providing vaccines for children will also improve the safety of other children who are too young to be immunized or individuals who cannot receive certain vaccines.

It is recommended that children receive 11 vaccinations before the age of six for Hepatitis B; rotavirus; Haemophilus influenzae type B; pneumococcal; poliovirus; influenza; varicella (chickenpox); Hepatitis A; meningococcal; measles, mumps, and rubella; and diphtheria, tetanus, and pertussis (whooping cough). Many of these immunizations are covered by most of the plans under the Affordable Care Act, including vaccines for Hepatitis A; Hepatitis B; influenza; meningococcal; pneumococcal; varicella; measles, mumps, and rubella; and diphtheria, tetanus, and pertussis.

Immunizations for Adults

All adults should receive an influenza vaccine every year, as well as a Tdap vaccine if they did not receive it as an adolescent. The Tdap vaccine prevents pertussis and should be administered each time a woman is pregnant, preferably between 27 and 36 weeks. All adults should also receive a Td booster every ten years to continuously prevent tetanus and diphtheria.

Additional adult vaccinations are recommended based on age, prior immunizations, health, lifestyle, occupation, and travel. Other factors, such as pregnancy, chronic illness, severe allergies, weak immune systems, and recent immunizations also determine whether adults should receive vaccines; therefore, it is important to discuss each vaccination with a medical professional.

Ingredients of Vaccines

Various chemicals are used in the production of vaccines, including: suspending fluid, such as sterile water, saline, or fluids with protein; preservatives and stabilizers, such as albumin, phenols, and glycine; adjuvants or enhancers to improve effectiveness; and small amount of the culture material used to grow the bacteria or virus that the vaccine is intended to prevent. However, it is important to realize that vaccines are safe and only small amounts of chemicals are added in order to preserve the vaccines and maintain their potency. The safety of vaccines is routinely monitored by government organizations and ingredients of the vaccine can be requested, as the immunization packaging details all ingredients and side effects of the vaccine.

Side Effects

Vaccinations are considered safe; however, there is always a risk of side effects when taking any medication. Common reactions to immunizations are soreness or redness around the injection site and a low-grade fever. Side effects to immunizations are usually mild and disappear within a few days. Some children may experience allergic reactions to a vaccine, but the reaction occurs very quickly after injection, typically while still in the doctor's office.

DATA AND ANALYSES

Data

Table 48.1 Comparison of 20th-century Annual Morbidity and Current Morbidity Rates of Vaccine-preventable Diseases: United States

Disease	20th-century annual morbidity	2010 reported cases	Percent reduction
Smallpox	29,005	0	100%
Diphtheria	21,053	0	100%
Pertussis	200,752	21,291	89%
Tetanus	580	8	99%
Polio (paralytic)	16,316	0	100%

(Continued)

Table 48.1 Comparison of 20th-century Annual Morbidity and Current Morbidity Rates of Vaccine-preventable Diseases: United States (*Continued*)

Disease	20th-century annual morbidity	2010 reported cases	Percent reduction
Measles	530,217	61	>99%
Mumps	162,344	2,528	98%
Rubella	47,745	6	>99%
Congenital rubella syndrome	152	0	100%
Haemophilus influenzae (<5 years of age)	20,000 (est.)	270	99%

Source: Centers for Disease Control and Prevention. 2011. "Epidemiology and Prevention of Vaccine-Preventable Diseases." Retrieved from: http://www.cdc.gov/vaccines/pubs/pinkbook/downloads/appendices/G/impact-of-vaccines.pdf

Analysis

Table 48.1 compares morbidity rates from the twentieth century and the year 2010 in order to examine the reduction of deaths due to vaccinations. For many diseases, such as smallpox, diphtheria, polio, and congenital rubella syndrome, vaccinations have prevented all related deaths. With zero reported deaths in 2010, the table presents that vaccinations are extremely important to preventing deaths related to the diseases above. All other diseases examined show high reduction rates as well, including pertussis, tetanus, measles, mumps, rubella, and Haemophilus influenzae in children under five years old. In total, vaccines reduced the morbidity rates by 1,004,000 individuals from the twentieth century to 2010. It is important to note, however, that this table does not represent how many individuals actually contracted these diseases—only the number who died from them. Other factors, such as greater technological advancement, may have had an impact on preventing deaths from these diseases.

Data

Table 48.2 Administered Influenza Vaccinations During the Past 12 Months, by Age Group and Sex: United States, 2012

Age	Percent of females	Percent of males	Average total
6 months to 4 years	53.2	56.6	54.9
5 years to 11 years	46.4	47.8	47.1
12 years to 17 years	36.2	35.3	35.7

Age	Percent of females	Percent of males	Average total
18 years to 49 years	30.3	22.2	26.3
50 years to 64 years	46.7	38.5	42.5
65 years and older	67.4	65.2	66.5

Source: Schiller, J.S., Ward, B.W., Freeman, G., & Peregoy, J.A. 2013. "Early release of selected estimates based on data from the 2012 National Health Interview Survey." National Center for Health Statistics. Retrieved from: http://www.cdc.gov/nchs/nhis.htm

Analysis

Table 48.2 presents a breakdown of influenza vaccinations that were administered throughout the year of 2012 by age group and sex. For both sexes combined, individuals 65 years and older received the most influenza vaccinations over the 12-month period, followed by children six months to four years old and 5–11 years old. For individuals six months and older and adults aged 18–64, females were more likely than males to receive the influenza vaccination. Individuals aged 18–49 years presented the lowest influenza vaccination rates, followed by 12–17-year-olds; however, it is recommended that an influenza vaccine is received each year for all individuals. Further research can examine why certain age groups are not receiving vaccinations and subsequent effects on the overall prevalence of vaccine-preventable diseases.

DISCUSSION QUESTIONS

1. Why isn't there a 100% reduction rate for deaths by all vaccine-preventable diseases? Do certain vaccines need to be altered to reach this goal or does it relate to the administration of the vaccine?
2. Why did measles, pertussis, and mumps contribute to the most deaths by vaccine-preventable diseases? Since the number of deaths related to measles was the highest during the twentieth century, why were deaths in 2010 reduced more than pertussis and mumps?
3. How do the morbidity rates of vaccine-preventable diseases in the United States relate to those in other countries? Are all of the same vaccines used worldwide to prevent these diseases?

4. Why do individuals 65 years and older account for the most influenza vaccinations in the United States? How can more younger individuals be educated about the importance of the vaccine?
5. Why do more females account for influenza vaccinations than males? What other factors relate to vaccination prevalence, such as race/ethnicity or income level?

49

VEGETARIAN AND VEGAN DIETS

INTRODUCTION

What Is a Vegetarian/Vegan?

Vegetarians and vegans are two similar, but slightly different, types of people. Both groups avoid meat products like pork and fish, usually citing both a desire to be healthier and a desire to reduce or end the inhumane treatment of animals. To replace the food they are no longer eating, both groups tend to eat more nuts, grains, and vegetables.

A vegetarian is someone who does not eat meat but does eat eggs and dairy products. Those looking to become vegan often start at this level to adapt to eating fewer animal products before stopping altogether.

A vegan is someone who does not eat any product that came from an animal. This is a more strict diet and often requires intense scrutiny to do successfully. Vegans often report weight loss, feeling healthier, and being less stressed as a result of their diet.

Benefits of These Lifestyles

There are many different positive aspects to being a vegetarian or vegan. For one, these diets often cost less, if done properly. Meat tends to be more expensive than tofu or similar nonmeat products, and can therefore help you save money. Vegetables are also full of fiber, which helps you feel full, meaning you do not have to buy as much food because you do not need to eat as much.

Moreover, many report feeling morally better about their food choices, since animals do not have to die to make the food they are buying. They also tend to buy free-range eggs and milk that came from "natural" cows as opposed to those given growth hormones to support this wholesome feeling. They will also avoid animal products like leather so that animals do not suffer to make any of their goods. By feeling less guilt over these decisions, vegetarians and vegans say they are more carefree and relaxed.

Some research suggests that avoiding meat increases a man's sex appeal, especially in respects to body odor. Children with high IQs are also more likely to turn to these diets at some point in their lives.

Also, vegetables, fruits, grains, and similar products are full of nutrients, ensuring you stay healthier. Vegetarians and vegans report that they are more relaxed and do not get sick as often as they did when eating meat, since they have stronger immune systems. Because meat can spoil easily or carry bacteria, those who follow these diets are also exposed to fewer diseases and bacteria. The nutrients and antioxidants also help you feel less stressed, which contributes to a generally healthier life.

In general, both of these diets are far better for you than meat-eating diets. The average American meat-eater has a cholesterol just over 200 while a vegan's is only around 130. Vegan diets can also increase the metabolism by up to 16%. Making this change also greatly lowers the risks of cancer, diabetes, obesity, heart disease, and many others. Elizabeth Blackburn, a noble prize winning researcher, found that a vegan diet could activate dormant DNA that prevents many short- and long-term diseases while deactivating those that cause serious illnesses. These alterations not only protect you, but your children as well, since active DNA is more likely to be passed on.

Downsides to Such Diets

Vegetarians and vegans are susceptible to vitamin deficiencies, despite the fact that vegetables and fruits are full of nutrients. They tend to be lacking in Omega-3 fatty acids, vitamin B12, calcium, vitamin D, iron, and other crucial supplements that help the body function. However, these deficiencies tend to affect those who remove meat from their diets without replacing them with other healthy food.

Also, the protein most vegetarians or vegans consume is incomplete. This means that the person will not be eating enough amino acids to build a complete protein, and this can lead to muscle loss or a slow metabolism. This is generally counteracted by combining amino acid sources, like by eating a salsa rich in corn and beans with a side of brown rice, or putting hummus on pita chips.

It can also be difficult to be a vegetarian or vegan at restaurants. Many soups are made with an animal stock, like chicken broth, and most dishes come with meat products as well. Even salads are often listed as containing cheese, many kinds of which are made with rennin, which comes from calf stomach, or have things like anchovies on top. It can be so difficult to eat out that many people on these diets simply choose not to do so.

DATA AND ANALYSES

Data

Table 49.1 Body Mass Index and Type 2 Diabetes Prevalence Related to Dietary Habits: United States, 2009

Dietary habit	Body mass index	Type 2 diabetes prevalence
Vegan	23.6	2.9%
Lacto-ovo-vegetarian	25.7	3.2%
Pesco-vegetarian	26.3	4.8%
Semi-vegetarian	27.3	6.1%
Nonvegetarian	28.8	7.6%

Source: Butler, T., Fraser, G.E., Tonstad, S., & Yan, R. 2009. "Type of vegetarian diet, body weight, and prevalence of type 2 diabetes." Retrieved from: http://www.ncbi.nlm.nih.gov/pubmed/19351712

Analysis

Table 49.1 presents body mass index (BMI) and type 2 diabetes prevalence related to dietary habits. In addition to there being a direct relationship between higher BMIs and type 2 diabetes prevalence, the dietary habits also had a direct impact on these statistics. The results show that individuals who are more restrictive with their dietary habits, cutting out meat, dairy, fish, and so forth present a lower BMI and type 2 diabetes prevalence. Nonvegetarians presented the highest average BMI at 28.8, as well as the highest type 2 diabetes prevalence at 7.6%. Meanwhile, vegan individuals who restrict all animal products presented the lowest average BMI at 23.6 and lowest type 2 diabetes prevalence at 2.9%. The healthy BMI range is between 18.5 and 24.9, while individuals whose BMI is 25 to 29.9 are considered overweight, and BMIs of 30 or greater are considered obese. These ranges support the findings that individuals who restrict all animal products are healthier than individuals with other dietary habits, as vegans were the only group who presented a healthy average BMI.

Data

Table 49.2 Mortality Rates Related to Dietary Habits: United States, 2009

Dietary habits	Deaths
Vegan	197
Lacto-ovo-vegetarian	815
Pesco-vegetarian	251
Semi-vegetarian	160
Nonvegetarian	1,147

Source: Beeson, W.L., Fan, J., Fraser, G.E., Jaceldo-Siegl, K., Knutsen, S., Orlich, M.J., Sabate, J., & Singh, P.N. 2013. "Vegetarian dietary patterns and mortality in Adventist health study 2." Retrieved from: http://www.ncbi.nlm.nih.gov/pubmed/23836264

Analysis

Table 49.2 presents mortality rates related to dietary habits, as found in the Adventist Health Study 2. Of 73,308 participants in the study, there was a total of 2,570 deaths during a mean follow-up time of 5.79 years. Results show that individuals who restrict all animal products as vegans present the lowest number of deaths at 197, while nonvegetarians present the highest number of deaths at 1,147. Evidently, there is a direct relationship between restricting animal products and a lower death rate; however, further research can apply this study to a wider range of participants, as well as determine the differences between types of vegetarians and their mortality rates. For example, further research can determine why lacto-ovo-vegetarians presented the second highest mortality rate, while semi-vegetarians presented the second lowest mortality rates. Lacto-ovo-vegetarians do not eat meat or fish, but consume dairy and egg products, while semi-vegetarians have a primarily plant-based diet, but occasionally consume meat products. These definitions provide a research question of whether consuming dairy and egg products raise mortality levels.

Data

Table 49.3 Reason for Choosing a Vegetarian Diet by Percent

Reason for becoming a vegetarian	Blank	No importance	Mildly important	Important	Very important
Animal rights	11.81	1.39	4.86	10.42	71.53
Environment	11.81	2.78	11.81	24.31	49.31
Health	12.5	2.78	14.58	22.22	47.92
Weight loss	13.89	32.64	20.14	15.28	18.06
Recommended by someone else	13.89	54.17	16.67	8.33	6.94

Source: http://www.advancedphysicalmedicine.org/blog/2011/11/04/the-anatomy-of-a-vegan/

Analysis

Table 49.3 breaks down a series of responses as to why people chose a vegetarian lifestyle, with the option to not respond available to all participants. The study overwhelmingly showed that animal rights was the most important factor in this decision, while being recommended to pursue it was the least important. Improving health and helping the environment were tied for importance; surprisingly, weight loss was viewed as substantially less important than overall health. This suggests that the moral impact of vegetarianism is more motivating than the physical and personal impact.

DISCUSSION QUESTIONS

1. Would you choose a vegetarian or vegan lifestyle? Why or why not (and which would you prefer)?
2. One major reason for people choosing a nonmeat lifestyle is to avoid cruelty to animals, but some studies suggest that the increase of these diets has not lowered the amount of animals killed for meat each year. How do you feel about this motivation, then? Is it effective? Could it be more effective? If so, how?
3. Nonmeat products can be produced faster and cheaper than meat products; considering this, do you believe enough is done to promote these lifestyles?

4. Do you believe there is enough education on vegetarian or vegan living? If not, what do you think should be done?
5. With life-threatening diseases and poverty on the rise, a non-meat diet offers more affordable food with long-term health benefits. Why do you think people avoid such diets, considering how helpful they can be?

50

VITAMIN CONSUMPTION AND SUPPLEMENTATION

INTRODUCTION

Understanding Vitamin Consumption/Supplementation

Vitamins refer to the organic compounds that are essential for the healthy growth, development, and functioning of the body throughout a person's lifetime. There are two types of vitamin nutrients: water-soluble vitamins and fat-soluble vitamins. While the body—namely, the kidneys—rids itself of excess amounts of the easily absorbed water-soluble vitamins, it stores amounts of fat-soluble vitamins for later use.

There are 13 vitamins, each of them either water soluble or fat soluble, that are absolutely essential for the human body to success-fully carry out its biological processes. Each with different functions ranging from red blood cell production to tooth and bone fortifica-tion, these 13 vitamins include:

- Vitamin A
- B vitamins, which is an umbrella term for these eight vitamins:
  - thiamine
  - riboflavin
  - niacin
  - pantothenic acid

  - biotin
  - vitamin B6
  - vitamin B12
  - folic acid
- Vitamin C
- Vitamin D
- Vitamin E
- Vitamin K

Consumption

The main source of vitamins is food. Every vitamin can be obtained through the consumption of fruits, vegetables, dairy products, and poultry, among other foods, that contain significant amounts of that specific vitamin. For example, vitamin C can be found in citrus fruits, vitamin A in carrots and spinach, and folic acid in leafy vegetables and grain products. Doctors recommend a balanced diet of a variety of foods to ensure sufficient amounts of the 13 essential vitamins.

Some vitamins can be obtained in other ways. For example, the body can obtain vitamin D by being exposed to sunlight and vitamin K by producing its own adequate supply.

Deficiency

Sometimes, a person cannot maintain a balanced diet; may be experiencing certain health problems; or is a vegetarian, vegan, pregnant, or breastfeeding. In any one of these cases, it is highly possible for there to be a shortage of essential vitamins in the body.

Although slight deficiencies may go unnoticed, prolonged and severe deficiencies can develop into serious health issues like anemia. Some of the symptoms of severe vitamin deficiency include:

- Weakness
- Fatigue
- Rapid heartbeat
- Labored breathing
- Easy bruising and bleeding
- Frequent nosebleeds
- Dry, splitting hair
- Cardiovascular disease
- Cancer

A doctor can easily diagnose a vitamin shortage with these symptoms, along with a blood test. A daily regimen of over-the-counter vitamin supplements is usually enough to help get the deficient vitamin levels under control, but a hospital stay may be necessary if the levels are especially low.

Negative Effects

Although vitamins are vital to nourishing the body and maintaining its health, they can be detrimental if they drastically exceed the recommended dietary allowance guidelines. Of course, every vitamin has its own specific consequences to health when taken in high dosages, but some of the main negative effects of taking in an excess of vitamins include:

- Nausea and vomiting
- Flushing and redness of skin
- Upset stomach
- Kidney stones
- Weakness
- Weight loss
- Dizziness
- Headaches
- Blurred vision
- Constipation

These can be exacerbated if accompanied by alcohol, medication, allergic reaction, or additional vitamin supplements. If a person experiences any of these effects, it is recommended for them to see a health care professional or visit an emergency room, depending on the severity of the symptoms.

DATA AND ANALYSES

Data

Table 50.1 Percentage of U.S. Men and Women Who Use Supplemental Vitamin D, by Age, 1988–2006

Gender/year	Age group		
Women	20–39 years old	40–59 years old	≥60 years old
1988–1994	30.3%	31.1%	29.7%
1999–2002	32.3%	45.1%	49.7%
2003–2006	33.8%	45.0%	56.3%

(Continued)

Table 50.1 Percentage of U.S. Men and Women Who Use Supplemental Vitamin D, by Age, 1988–2006 (*Continued*)

Gender/year	Age group		
Men	20–39 years old	40–59 years old	≥60 years old
1988–1994	22.2%	26.0%	23.7%
1999–2002	26.4%	34.7%	38.1%
2003–2006	26.5%	38.0%	44.0%

Source: http://www.cdc.gov/nchs/data/databriefs/db61.htm#dietary

Analysis

Table 50.1 provides an interesting timeline of men and women aged 20 and over who take supplemental vitamin D. The data not only takes into account three time frames (1988–1994, 1999–2002, and 2003–2006), it also considers three age groups of participants of the study (20–39 years old, 40–59 years old, and 60 years or older).

Although this data applies to supplemental vitamin D, it is worth noting that general supplement use has been on the rise since 1998 among adults over 20 years old—a fact into which this data provides additional and valuable insight.

For each of the three age groups surveyed, the percentage of men and women taking supplemental vitamin D significantly increased from 1988 to 2006. The most significant change was found in adults 60 years and older. For example, 29.7% of women in the 1988–1994 time period took supplemental vitamin D, while 56.3% did in the 2003–2006 time period. Similarly, 23.7% of men in the 1988–1994 time period took supplemental vitamin D, while 44.0% did in the 2003–2006 time period. Overall, women had higher percentages than men in both age and year categories.

Data

Table 50.2 Percentage of U.S. Population Who Reported Taking Multivitamin/minerals in a Given Month, by Age, 2003–2006

Age group	Men	Women
1–3 years	27%	25%
4–8 years	35%	28%
9–13 years	18%	23%
14–18 years	14%	19%
19–30 years	25%	30%
31–50 years	32%	38%

Age group	Men	Women
51–70 years	40%	48%
≥71 years	43%	48%

Note: In this data, "multivitamin/mineral" is defined as products containing at least three vitamins and at least one mineral.

Source: http://ods.od.nih.gov/factsheets/MVMS-HealthProfessional/#en1

Analysis

Table 50.2 shows the percentage of men and women of different age groups consuming multivitamin/minerals. During the 2003–2006 period, it was found that the older a person, the higher their consumption percentage was. For example, men and women aged 71 years or older yielded percentages larger (43% and 48%, respectively) than those in the one-to-three-year age group (27% and 25%, respectively). Interestingly, more men took multivitamins/minerals before the 9–13 age group, at which point women dominated percentage-wise.

Data

Table 50.3 Recommended Dietary Allowance for Vitamin C in Milligrams per Day, 2000

Life stage	Recommended milligrams per day
Birth to 6 months	40
Infants 7–12 months	50
Children 1–3 years	15
Children 4–8 years	25
Children 9–13 years	45
Teen boys 14–18 years	75
Teen girls 14–18 years	65
Adult men ≥19 years	90
Adult women ≥19 years	75
Pregnant women	85
Breastfeeding women	120
Smokers	+35 to corresponding age

Source: http://ods.od.nih.gov/factsheets/VitaminC-QuickFacts/

Analysis

Table 50.3 outlines the recommended dietary allowance for just one of many vitamins, vitamin C, in milligrams per day. Babies and adults need the highest intake of vitamin C. Adult men aged 19 or over need about 90 mg of vitamin C daily. This is more than adult women aged 19 or over, who need about 75 mg/day. Breastfeeding women need the most out of those listed (120 mg/day), while children aged one to three years need the least (15 mg/day).

DISCUSSION QUESTIONS

1. Although there are 13 essential vitamins, other vitamins do exist. What are some other vitamins that you know of and how do they help the body?
2. Vitamins are meant to help the body grow and maintain health, but too much of a certain vitamin can have dangerous effects on the body. What other substances have you learned about that can be detrimental if taken in excess?
3. According to Table 50.1, there has been in increase in the use of supplemental vitamin D over the course of almost two decades. What are some possible reasons for this?
4. With a deficiency of most vitamins, like vitamins B and D, it becomes much easier for a person to bruise their skin or bleed. Why do you think this occurs?
5. According to Table 50.3, breastfeeding women have a significantly higher daily allowance of vitamin C than pregnant women and women who are neither pregnant nor breastfeeding. What are some possible reasons why a breastfeeding woman might need more vitamin C?

RESOURCES FOR FURTHER RESEARCH

Academy for Eating Disorders. (n.d.). Retrieved June 29, 2014, from http://www.aedweb.org

Adolescent pregnancy. (2011). National Institutes of Health, Medline Plus. Retrieved June 29, 2014, from http://www.nlm.nih.gov/medlineplus/ency/article/001516.htm

Allergic reactions: tips to remember. (2013). American Academy of Allergy, Asthma & Immunology. Retrieved June 29, 2014, from http://www.aaaai.org/conditions-and-treatments/library/at-a-glance/allergic-reactions.aspx

Allergies. (2013). Mayo Clinic. Retrieved June 29, 2014, from http://www.mayoclinic.org/diseases-conditions/allergies/basics/symptoms/con-20034030

American Cancer Society. (n.d.). *Breast cancer.* American Cancer Society. Retrieved June 29, 2014, from http://www.cancer.org/cancer/breastcancer/detailedguide/breast-cancer-detailed-guide-toc

American Psychiatric Association. (2013). *Diagnostic and statistical manual of mental disorders* (5th ed.). Arlington, VA: American Psychiatric Publishing.

Anemia. (2013). Mayo Clinic. Retrieved June 29, 2014, from http://www.mayoclinic.org/diseases-conditions/anemia/basics/definition/con-20026209

Anorexia nervosa and related eating disorders. (n.d.). Retrieved June 29, 2014, from http://www.anred.com

Autoimmune disorders. (2011). National Institutes of Health. Retrieved June 29, 2014, from http://www.nlm.nih.gov/medlineplus/ency/article/000816.htm

Benaroch, R. (2012). *Children's vaccines.* WebMD. Retrieved June 29, 2014, from http://www.webmd.com/children/vaccines/immunizations-vaccines-power-of-preparation?page=3

Benoist, B., Cogswell, M., Egli, I., & McLean, E. (2008). *Worldwide prevalence of anaemia 1993–2005.* World Health Organization. Retrieved June 29, 2014, from http://whqlibdoc.who.int/publications/2008/9789241596657_eng.pdf

Breast reconstruction. (2012). National Institutes of Health, National Cancer Institute. Retrieved June 29, 2014, from http://www.cancer.gov/cancertopics/wyntk/breast/page7

Butler, P. (2014). *Anemia overview.* United States Securities and Exchange Commission: 71–74. Retrieved June 29, 2014, from http://www.sec.gov/Archives/edgar/data/1517022/000119312514055104/d629509ds1.htm

Centers for Disease Control and Prevention. (2014). *Heart disease.* Retrieved from http://www.cdc.gov/heartdisease/

Colorectal cancer risk by age. (2013). Centers for Disease Control and Prevention Division of Cancer Prevention and Control. Retrieved June 29, 2014, from http://www.cdc.gov/cancer/colorectal/statistics/age.htm

Digestive diseases. (2014). National Institutes of Health. Retrieved June 29, 2014, from http://www.nlm.nih.gov/medlineplus/digestivediseases.html

The Eating Disorder Foundation. (n.d.). Retrieved June 29, 2014, from http://www.eatingdisorderfoundation.org

Eating Disorders Coalition. (n.d.). Retrieved June 29, 2014, from http://www.eatingdisorderscoalition.org

Evaluating health information. (2014). National Institutes of Health. Retrieved June 22, 2014, from http://www.nlm.nih.gov/medlineplus/evaluatinghealthinformation.html

Everhart, J.E. (2008). *The burden of digestive diseases in the United States.* National Institutes of Health. Retrieved June 29, 2014, from http://www.niddk.nih.gov/about-niddk/strategic-plans-reports/Pages/burden-digestive-diseases-in-united-statesreport.aspx#Index

Fact sheet on stress. (2014). National Institute of Mental Health. Retrieved June 29, 2014, from http://www.nimh.nih.gov/health/publications/stress/index.shtml

Facts about birth defects. (2014). Centers for Disease Control and Prevention. Retrieved June 29, 2014, from http://www.cdc.gov/ncbddd/birthdefects/facts.html

Foodborne illness, foodborne disease (sometimes called "food poisoning"). (2012). Centers for Disease Control and Prevention Food Safety Office.

Retrieved June 29, 2014, from http://www.cdc.gov/foodsafety/facts.html

Getting pregnant. (2013). Mayo Clinic. Retrieved June 29, 2014, from http://www.mayoclinic.org/symptoms-of-pregnancy/ART-20043853?p=1

Goodman, J. (2010). *Cancer deaths vs. cancer research.* National Center for Policy Analysis. Retrieved June 29, 2014, from http://healthblog.ncpa.org/cancer-deaths-vs-cancer-research/

Health effects of cigarette smoking. (2014). Centers for Disease Control and Prevention Office on Smoking and Health, National Center for Chronic Disease Prevention and Health Promotion. Retrieved June 29, 2014, from http://www.cdc.gov/tobacco/data_statistics/fact_sheets/health_effects/effects_cig_smoking/

Heart disease. (2013). Mayo Clinic. Retrieved from http://www.mayo-clinic.org/diseases-conditions/heart-disease/basics/symptoms/con-20034056

Hudson, J.I., Hiripi, E., Pope, H.G., & Kessler, R.C. (2007). *The prevalence and correlates of eating disorders in the National Comorbidity Survey Replication.* National Institute of Mental Health. Retrieved June 29, 2014, from http://www.nimh.nih.gov

Incidence, prevalence, and cost of sexually transmitted infections in the United States. (2013). Centers for Disease Control and Prevention. Retrieved June 29, 2014, from http://www.cdc.gov/std/stats/sti-estimates-fact-sheet-feb-2013.pdf

Infant mortality. (2013). Centers for Disease Control and Prevention. Retrieved June 29, 2014, from http://www.cdc.gov/reproductive-health/maternalinfanthealth/infantmortality.htm

John Hopkins Medicine. (2014). *Digestive disorders.* Retrieved June 29, 2014, from http://www.hopkinsmedicine.org/healthlibrary/conditions/adult/digestive_disorders/digestive_disorders_home_85,P00385/

Krucik, J., & Roddick, G. (2012). *Autoimmune disease.* Healthline Networks. Retrieved June 29, 2014, from http://www.healthline.com/health/autoimmune-disorders

Labor and delivery, postpartum care. (2012). Mayo Clinic. Retrieved June 29, 2014, from http://www.mayoclinic.org/c-section-recovery/ART-20047310?p=1

MedlinePlus. (2014). *Allergy.* National Institutes of Health. Retrieved June 29, 2014, from http://www.nlm.nih.gov/medlineplus/allergy.html#cat5

Miniño, A.M., & Klein, R.J. (2007). *Mortality from major cardiovascular diseases: United States, 2007.* Centers for Disease Control and Prevention. Retrieved from http://www.cdc.gov/nchs/data/hestat/cardio2007/cardio2007.htm

Murphy, S.L., Xu, J., & Kochanek, M.A. (2010). *Deaths: final data for 2010.* National Vital Statistics Report. Retrieved June 29, 2014, from http://www.cdc.gov/nchs/fastats/anemia.htm

National Association of Anorexia Nervosa and Associated Disorders. (n.d.). Retrieved June 29, 2014, from http://www.anad.org

National Eating Disorders Association. (n.d.). Retrieved June 29, 2014, from http://www.nationaleatingdisorders.org

Physical activity guidelines for Americans. (2008). U.S. Department of Health & Human Services. Retrieved from http://www.health .gov/paguidelines/guidelines

Preterm birth. (2013). Centers for Disease Control and Prevention. Retrieved June 29, 2014, from http://www.cdc.gov/reproductivehealth/ maternalinfanthealth/pretermbirth.htm

Risk & protective factors. (2014). U.S. Department of Health & Human Services Office of Adolescent Health. Retrieved June 29, 2014, from http:// www.hhs.gov/ash/oah/adolescent-health-topics/substance-abuse/tobacco/risk-and-protective-factors.html

Sexually transmitted disease surveillance 2011. (2012). Centers for Disease Control and Prevention Division of STD Prevention. Retrieved June 29, 2014, from http://wonder.cdc.gov/wonder/help/STD/STD-Surv2011.pdf

Sexually transmitted diseases (STDs). (2013). Mayo Clinic. Retrieved June 29, 2014, from http://www.mayoclinic.org/diseases-conditions/sexually-transmitted-diseases-stds/basics/definition/ con-20034128

Smoking. (2014). National Institutes of Health, MedlinePlus. Retrieved June 29, 2014, from http://www.nlm.nih.gov/medlineplus/ smoking.html

STD trends in the United States. (2013). Centers for Disease Control and Prevention. Retrieved June 29, 2014, from http://www.cdc.gov/std/ stats11/trends-2011.pdf

Stress—introduction. (2010). HealthCentral. Retrieved June 29, 2014, from http://www.healthcentral.com/ency/408/guides/000031_1. html?ic=506019

Sudden infant death syndrome. (2014). Centers for Disease Control and Prevention. Retrieved June 29, 2014, from http://www.cdc.gov/SIDS/ INDEX.HTM

Thyroid cancer. (2014). American Cancer Society. Retrieved June 29, 2014, from http://www.cancer.org/cancer/thyroidcancer/ detailedguide/thyroid-cancer-what-is-thyroid-cancer

Thyroid cancer. (2014). Mayo Clinic. Retrieved June 29, 2014, from http:// www.mayoclinic.org/diseases-conditions/thyroid-cancer/basics/ treatment/con-20043551

Tobacco-related mortality. (2014). Centers for Disease Control and Prevention Office on Smoking and Health, National Center for Chronic Disease Prevention and Health Promotion. Retrieved June 29, 2014, from http://www.cdc.gov/tobacco/data_statistics/fact_sheets/ health_effects/tobacco_related_mortality/

Understanding anemia—the basics. (n.d.). WebMD. Retrieved June 29, 2014, from http://www.webmd.com/a-to-z-guides/understanding-anemia-basics?page=2

What is a cesarean delivery? (2012). National Institutes of Child Health and Human Development. Retrieved June 29, 2014, from http://www.nichd.nih.gov/health/topics/pregnancy/conditioninfo/Pages/cesarean.aspx

What is anemia? (2012). U.S. Department of Health & Human Services, National Heart, Lung, and Blood Institute. Retrieved June 29, 2014, from http://www.nhlbi.nih.gov/health/health-topics/topics/anemia/

What is attention deficit hyperactivity disorder (ADHD, ADD)? (n.d.). U.S. Department of Health & Human Services, National Institute of Mental Health. Retrieved June 29, 2014, from http://www.nimh.nih.gov/health/topics/attention-deficit-hyperactivity-disorder-adhd/index.shtml